A Gift for Healing

A Gift *for* Healing

How to Use
Therapeutic
Touch

DEBORAH COWENS, M.S.N., R.N., A.N.P.

with TOM MONTE

Crown Trade Paperbacks   New York

Published by Crown Trade Paperbacks, 201 East 50th Street, New York, New York 10022. Member of the Crown Publishing Group.

Random House, Inc. New York, Toronto, London, Sydney, Auckland
http://www.randomhouse.com/
Crown Trade Paperbacks and colophon are trademarks of Crown Publishers, Inc.

Design by June Bennett-Tantillo

Printed in the United States of America

Library of Congress Cataloging-in-Publication Data

Cowens, Deborah.
A gift for healing : how to use therapeutic touch / Deborah Cowens and Tom Monte.
p.   cm.
Includes index.
1. Touch—Therapeutic use.   I. Monte, Tom.   II. Title.
RZ999.C83   1996
615.8′9—dc20   96-4102
CIP

ISBN 0-517-88651-0 (pbk.)

10   9   8   7   6   5   4   3   2   1

First Edition

This book is dedicated to all the students of energy work and to all our patients who teach us.

Author's Note

It is my hope that you, the reader, will be able to raise your inherent gift for healing by using the techniques put forth in this book. Remember, your learning and growth are a journey that is not completed in one reading. Take time to do each of the exercises. Provide the space and time to allow yourself to grow with the process. As you are patient with your clients, be patient with yourself in your learning.

This book is intended to complement, and not replace or substitute for, the medical advice of physicians. Before commencing any healing touch therapy, the patient should have a thorough physical by a doctor.

The case histories are real and are presented as accurately as possible. All names and identifying characteristics of people and places have been changed to assure their anonymity.

Contents

Acknowledgments

I wish to acknowledge with love all my family, especially David, Meghan, and Samantha, for all their support for me through this process.

In addition, I would like to thank Joyce, Doris, Linda, Phyllis, Sandy, and Connie, without whose advice, encouragement, and typing I would have faltered.

A special thanks to Clark Godfrey, Betty Taylor Godfrey, and Emily Osman for their artistic input.

Illustrations

'Tis the human touch in this world that counts,
The touch of your hand and mine

FROM *THE HUMAN TOUCH*
BY SPENCER MICHAEL FREE

Introduction

Therapeutic touch is perhaps the first form of health care ever utilized. Every parent since Adam and Eve has used this practice instinctively when he or she has placed a loving hand on a child to reduce discomfort, help heal a wound, or alleviate a fever. Therapeutic touch is the most human of all forms of healing, using the hands to reach out in service to another person in a gesture of peace, balance, and love.

This book is meant to teach you how to help yourself and others—your family, friends, and loved ones—overcome disorders of the body, mind, or spirit. You do not have to have any special knowledge or expertise to learn or utilize this practice effectively. All you need is provided in the pages that follow. People who practice therapeutic touch regularly will find its power to heal remarkable, and sometimes even miraculous. My intention for this book is that it help people directly and also that it serves as a bridge between two worlds of healing: the modern and the alternative forms of medicine. I would like doctors and other health professionals to understand therapeutic touch so that they can begin to utilize it in hospitals and medical practices. By providing you, the reader, and, perhaps, the patient with information that will give you a real understanding and confidence in the efficacy of therapeutic touch, I hope to help you begin to take part in your own healing and take charge of your own health. By educating yourself in this healing art and seeing its effectiveness, you will be part of a grass-roots influencing of the medical profession. For these reasons, I have deliberately tried to keep this book practical and simple, without oversimplifying or doing an injustice to the traditional and ancient philosophies that underlie the practice.

I do not intend for this book to replace or substitute for medical advice or intervention. Healing touch should be used in conjunction with conventional medical therapies. Because healing touch relaxes the body and triggers the body's self-healing energies, it increases the effectiveness of medicines and other treatments.

I became a practitioner of healing touch after traveling a long, circuitous path that led me into both orthodox medicine and alternative healing. I have bachelor's and master's degrees in nursing, an advanced degree in nutrition, and I'm a certified nurse practitioner, which means that I am licensed to prescribe medication and to treat patients independently while under the supervision of a medical doctor. On the other hand, I am a certified herbalist and have a formal training in therapeutic touch. Also, I have studied a wide range of holistic or traditional healing practices, such as Chinese medicine. This dual path in conventional and traditional medicine unfolded in a series of decisions that seemed at the time to be motivated chiefly by my immediate needs and desires. But looking back over the past twenty years at the myriad subjects I studied and the very different teachers with whom I studied, all seem so orderly now, as if my education was designed to get me precisely to the place I now find myself: a practitioner of modern and ancient medicine.

Getting Here from There

I was born and raised in Verona, New York, and ever since I was twelve or thirteen years old, I knew that I wanted to go into medicine. At first, I thought I would be a doctor, but my father dissuaded me. Medicine isn't really a good profession for women, he advised me. You're better off going into nursing or teaching, he said. This was the 1950s, and the world was different then, with both sexes locked into a worldview that seems archaic to most of us today. My father was looking out for me, and advised me according to how he saw things. I didn't realize it at the time, but he was actually helping me make the right choice, though he might have been influenced, at least in part, by some rather dated reasons. In any case, I have been thanking him for years for guiding me correctly.

My parents were conscious of the importance of eating healthful, good-quality food. We ate organic vegetables that my father grew in his garden and organic chicken and beef raised on my grandmother's farm. Healthy food and attitudes were an important part of my and my three siblings' upbringing.

While very traditional in some ways, my parents also possessed unique and special talents. My mother seemed to have a sixth sense about people. She had insight into their behavior and motives; she could perceive people's feelings that existed below the surface, sometimes even before they could articulate such feelings themselves. This ability was apparent to people, and many of my mother's friends and family came regularly to ask her advice.

My mother was also a wonderful dressmaker. She could take a pattern into a fabric store, look at five bolts of material, and visualize how the dress would look when made from those five different cloths. This visual ability extended to other areas of life, such as how a room would look if it were redecorated. I realized later that my mother had a highly developed ability to visualize, or mentally "see," three-dimensionally. My father had a similar trait. He was an industrial arts teacher and a carpenter and could make just about anything out of wood. Often, he would work without a schematic and produce the most beautiful furniture, cabinets, and other wood objects. These abilities were inherited by all four of their children—my brother, two sisters, and me. All of us talked about feelings—our own and others'—and could hold an image in our minds and discuss it at length without any sense that we were doing anything extraordinary.

After graduation from high school, I studied nursing at Niagara University, where, among other things, I was trained to be a keen observer. One of my teachers in medical-surgical nursing would bring us into the waiting room of our hospital and train us to observe and understand patients. She would insist that we ask ourselves specific questions that would open and expand our perceptions of people and situations. "What did you feel about the person you talked to?" she would ask. "What could you tell about the people you observed?" "What was the patient going through?" "What symptoms of disease did she or he exhibit?" And so forth.

During one of my early classes, which was held in the hospital wards, I witnessed how intuitive my instructor was about people. She asked us to list the things we observed about the patients we encountered as we followed her on her rounds that morning. We went into a patient's room with her and observed as she held the patient's hand, said "Good morning," and asked three questions: "How are you today?" "How did you sleep?" "How is your pain?" Everyone wrote down three or four sentences about what they had observed. When our teacher revealed what she had observed, it amounted to two pages of writing. Even more remarkable, she had gotten all of that information merely by holding the person's hand. I was amazed. I knew right then that I wanted to be able to touch like that—to feel a human being so deeply that I could discern his or her inner state merely by holding his or her hand.

During my senior year, I worked at Roswell Park, the cancer institute in Buffalo. The instructor and the nurses on the floor were wonderful in their teaching and guidance. In this place my ability to touch people on many levels began to develop. One patient, an elderly woman, had been hospitalized for a gynecological cancer that had spread to her bones. She was in great pain and was about to undergo gynecological surgery. Her doctors did not hold out much hope for her recovery, however. In those days, nurses still prepared patients for surgery by removing the hair from their abdomen with a razor, and I had to do this for this woman. After about five minutes, she began crying, both because of the pain the shaving caused and because of her fear of dying. I stopped shaving her and instinctively put my hands on the place where she had the most pain. Meanwhile, I said a prayer that the pain would be relieved. After a few minutes, she told me that she felt better and we could continue the shaving. Periodically, she asked me to stop, and I would have to put my hand on her stomach to relieve the pain. At this point, I had no awareness of therapeutic touch. I touched her instinctively and with the singular intention of relieving her discomfort.

During my senior year, I rotated into psychiatric practice, where I encountered Bertha, a woman in her sixties who went around the ward using her finger as an imaginary gun and shooting at make-believe beings. I asked my instructor for advice on how to deal with Bertha. "Mimic her in order to understand better what she may be feeling," my teacher advised. From that point on, I started to mimic Bertha's behavior. Once, while doing just that, I nearly knocked over a lamp, and as I righted it, I confessed to Bertha that I felt silly shooting at imaginary people. Bertha looked me straight in the eye and with utter lucidity said, "Well, you look silly." The other patients who were standing nearby all looked at me and nodded their agreement and then smiled. I laughed, and for the next four weeks, Bertha and I were friends. For a while, she appeared perfectly sane to me—that is, until I told her that I would be cycling out of that part of the hospital. Upon hearing the news, Bertha shut me out and resumed shooting her imaginary enemies. She seemed as psychotic as ever. But the experience taught me that health and illness are locked in a battle within us all, and that no matter how ill a person may be, there is always a degree of health within, as well. That healthy aspect of the patient is the part that a healer seeks to strengthen in the patient's struggle to overcome disease.

From Niagara, I went on to graduate school to work with emotionally disturbed children. Behind all my studies was a deep desire to find the root causes of disease. I always believed that if I could find the cause, I could somehow pull the disease out by its roots. After graduation, I worked at Rome City Hospital, in New York State, as a graduate nurse for three months, and then went to Boston University, where I received a master's degree in child psychiatric nursing, which made me a clinical specialist. I practiced for three years in child psychiatry and also taught in a nursing school.

As a nurse, I learned quickly how the power of touch helped my patients. Whenever I held patients' hands, or rubbed their backs, the effect was most powerful and obvious. They relaxed. Gradually, fear diminished. The patient trusted me more and felt more comfortable with what lay ahead. It's remarkable how much safety is communicated simply by touching a person. Is this why we instinctively touch our children to reassure them? I wondered.

In 1972, I worked at Boston University's Child Guidance Center and Infant Development Unit, which later became Solomon Carter Fuller Mental Health Center. I worked with families in lower socioeconomic brackets. Many of the mothers in this group gave birth to premature babies, many of whom died. The infant mortality rate was exceedingly high. These preemies were often placed in the neonatal intensive care unit, where they were kept on life-support systems. Their mothers were often afraid of all the machines. That fear created a kind of wall between the mother and her baby.

One of the practices I instituted was to get the mothers to touch and stroke their babies for extended periods of time. This helped the mothers overcome their fear of the machines. Even more importantly, the stroking helped the children to develop far more rapidly and thus lowered the risk of premature death. We worked directly with the infants, too, many of whom were deformed. We started passive exercise programs that resulted in remarkable improvement in their development of motor skills and coordination.

Premature babies are often no bigger than a small fist and far more shriveled than the fingers of an old man. They are vulnerable and delicate. Yet there is something that emanates from these tiny, vulnerable infants that I can only describe as radiant energy. You feel it when you touch such an infant or place your hand near her body. As your hand gets within a few inches of the child's head or back, you can feel a certain energy coming off her body. Your hand tells you something is there, but you cannot see it. At first, I wasn't really sure what I was sensing. The only thing I could call it then was "spirit" or "energy." Since I had no training in these areas, such words made me uncomfortable. I could find no rational place for my perceptions.

Anyone who has ever worked with children will tell you that the experience is transformative. One of the things you learn is that a child's view of life is radically different from an adult's. Children are thrilled to have you near and are very open to your touch. They don't have the same defensive or skeptical walls around them that adults have. Children let you in. I began to wonder if this high degree of receptivity, openness, and acceptance actually enhanced the healing process, because, despite their obvious vulnerability, children often make the most miraculous recoveries against incredible odds.

A few years later in my career, I became fascinated by the effects of diet on health. At age twenty-nine, I entered nutrition school to learn about holistic health and nutrition. I also realized that nutrition was an area that all of us could control, to some extent, and therefore gave us the power to heal ourselves. This idea resonated with me, in part because of the food I ate as a child. At that time, the organic and natural foods movement started to pick up steam.

At nutrition school, I began to realize that I possessed a certain degree of extrasensory perception that gave me insight into a person's inner condition. I discovered that when I looked at someone with the intention of understanding his health, I could sometimes perceive certain events taking place within the person's body—and even his organs. When I touched the area where a patient's liver is or lay my hands on his abdomen, I would get an image of the inner condition and whether or not the person suffered from some form of physical or emotional pathology. I also started to concentrate and pray while touching patients. Very often, the person would tell me that his or her pain or inflammation had noticeably diminished with my touch. This recognition profoundly altered my life. It also gave my previous experiences with touch far greater meaning.

In 1982, I went to the healing and educational center Interface, in Boston, for training in therapeutic touch. I knew right away that this approach was right for me. It was as if all my training and so many of my experiences had already formed the foundation for this work. I had been prepared, so the minute I walked into that classroom, nothing that was taught seemed odd, or bizarre, or in any way out of the ordinary realm of human experience. The training also gave me a language to describe my feelings and experiences, as well as a set of techniques to use in my practice.

Afterward, I actively sought spiritual experience and instruction and learned some of the healing methods of Native Americans—including those involving therapeutic touch. I am particularly grateful for my ongoing study with Oh Shinnah Fastwolf, an Apache, and Twylah Nitsch, a Seneca. These two Native American women supported and encouraged me; each gave me a more holistic worldview through the Native American understanding of life. They taught me how to do energy work, how to shape my intent, how to use imagery to heal, and to learn patience with myself as I proceed through my own life journey. Oh Shinnah taught me the importance of using ritual and prayer, not only to become more receptive to healing energy but to keep focused during the process. Twylah helped me with my technique. But more importantly, she stressed patience and the need for me to remember who I am. Twylah maintains that each of us, on an unconscious level, possesses all knowledge, including the knowledge of our own personal spiritual identity. Learning is actually remembering, and the ultimate memory is to recognize your true spiritual self.

I try to convey to you the essence and practice of all these teachings in this book. As we journey together through it, I hope you will learn how to enhance your healing abilities and your extrasensory perception so that you can help yourself and others. Some chapters will contain exercises that will help you focus your energies as you learn healing touch.

Healing Begins with Respect and Faith

During my many years of study, I have witnessed and helped to bring about many remarkable recoveries, as I will report throughout the pages of this book. I also learned ways of understanding and sensing the energy body, or life force, that exists around all people. But what my teachers gave me first was the right attitude for approaching this practice. The healer doesn't heal; he or she facilitates a process that is active and implicit within all of us. The seeds of healing exist in the person in search of help. It is important that the recipient of healing touch be open and respectful of this healing process. In a certain sense, we must be like children—open, receptive, and ready to learn. By maintaining an open mind and spirit, the recipient allows the energy that flows to him or her to be taken in and utilized efficiently.

A reverential attitude toward the healing process is the basis of all traditional healing approaches, and still is throughout the world. Healing is not seen as a lucky mix of chemical processes in most cultures, but is considered an expression of the harmonious joining of heaven and earth. Healing rituals are practiced in many cultures to evoke greater faith, which in turn triggers the healing forces within the person who is seeking help and within his family and community.

The scientific studies from which I report that prove the efficacy of therapeutic touch show that people benefit from healing touch no matter what they believe. My experience has shown, however, that those who are more open and receptive make quicker progress. For this reason, I always maintain that *healing is a gift you give yourself,* because you must receive this enhanced life energy and allow your body, mind, and spirit to utilize it for whatever purpose you need. You marshal these enhanced energies for your own purposes. Something inside of you accepts and embraces the healing process.

As Norman Cousins wrote in *Anatomy of an Illness:* "Drugs are not always necessary. Belief in recovery always is."

We live in a time when bridges between orthodox and alternative medicine must be built if we are to have a truly humane and effective health care system. Medicine and health care are now in the throes of a revolution. Today, more and more people are seeking the counsel and treatment of alternative medical practitioners of acupuncture, massage therapies, herbalism, diet, and other traditional healing methods. Healing touch is among those practices gaining credibility with both the lay public and medical professionals. Indeed, Western society's worldview is changing dramatically as science proves the wisdom and the efficacy of ancient healing approaches. This trend will continue as more and more people seek creative ways of healing old and intractable disorders. I hope that this book, *A Gift for Healing,* will inspire people to utilize this practice and in the process embrace a larger understanding of healing—and themselves.

Part One

Learning the Language of Energy

1

⚛

The Science of an Ancient Art

A healing power flows from your hands.

This power can help people overcome sickness, negative beliefs, and old and useless habits. It can heal wounds, reduce pain, boost energy, improve psychological health, and help to manage and heal chronic illness. Healing touch, or what has been known in the West as the "laying on of hands," has been used as a medical treatment technique in virtually every traditional culture. Healing touch can also serve as a powerful adjunct to conventional medical therapy. Today, scientific studies consistently prove its power to heal, though researchers still don't understand how or why the practice works.

In the broadest sense, healing touch is the act of consciously directing life energy from its infinite source, through the practitioner, to the person in need of assistance. It is done with the specific intention of giving love, support, and help in overcoming a physical or psychological problem. This conscious transfer of energy can be facilitated and enhanced through an assortment of techniques and by deepening your understanding of the practice.

Today, healing or therapeutic touch is being taught in eighty colleges and universities in the United States and is being utilized by medical professionals around the country. My own profession of nursing is the leader in this movement, in large part because nurses traditionally offer emotional support, including solace and compassion, often in the form of touching. For all practitioners of healing touch, the practice has become an outgrowth of our desire to help people in times of crisis or pain.

To understand the *how* and the *why* of healing touch so that we can utilize its therapeutic value, we must open up to a larger view of ourselves and of life. In a sense, we must go beyond the restricted definition of life that is imposed upon us by our modern culture. We must view our lives in a more traditional way—that is, in the way people have seen life through most of human history: as a physical, emotional, and spiritual whole connected to other lives and to the greater life of our natural environment.

We must also view health in a similar way. Rather than seeing health as merely the absence of symptoms, we must see it in a larger context—again, as a condition of wholeness or integration of body, mind, and spirit within the greater cultural and natural environment. Each of us represents a vast potential to grow and develop emotionally, psychologically, and spiritually. Our world demands such growth and development. Indeed, our health may be predicated on our ability to reach down continually into the psyche and bring forth and develop the unique skills and characteristics that lie deep within us. Yet, few of us realize our potential, in part because many of our better characteristics are hidden within us, repressed or denied by fears and false beliefs. These repressive emotions act as walls of energy or blockages between our potential or true self and our own conscious minds. Thus, we confront the world with only parts of our character, strength, and spirit available to us.

Besides preventing self-realization and self-understanding, energetic barriers can also block life energy from flowing through the body. In the traditional model of health, the entire body—and each of its parts—depends upon the optimal flow of life energy to function properly. When barriers to the life force deprive certain parts of the body of life energy, these cells, organs, and tissues consequently become weak, sluggish, and stagnant, and gradually degenerate. With time, these conditions can bring on some form of disease. The illness may be called one name or another, but the true underlying source of the physical or mental problem is a diminution of the life force flowing to that particular part of the body. Therefore, deep healing begins by a restoration of the life force to areas of the body that are deprived of life energy.

Healing touch can assist us in dealing with all of these issues by removing the blockages, or repressive barriers, that prevent energy from flowing. Thus, it can restore energy to parts of the body deprived of life force. In the same way, healing touch can help us arrive at a deeper self-understanding and lead to a fuller expression of those talents and the creativity that lie within us.

After a single session of healing touch, the recipient invariably feels refreshed, stronger, and clearer, as if he or she has just had a very restful nap. With repeated sessions, the health effects of healing touch are remarkable. Acute physical symptoms and long-standing chronic complaints are reduced or disappear.

The psychological and spiritual transformation is equally impressive. Gradually, the blockages that have kept the person from experiencing and understanding himself or herself are removed from the energy field, and hence from the person's life. Old, restrictive beliefs are shed like a skin that the person has outgrown. The person lets go of illness-inducing behavior patterns and sees more clearly how to live in more health-promoting ways.

One of the goals of healing touch is to help people become more aware of who they truly are and incorporate that awareness into daily life in practical ways. I call this "expanded integrated awareness." Only by grounding that awareness in practical daily activities can any of us truly integrate ourselves. With time, we free ourselves from self-limiting attitudes and develop a healthier and much greater picture of who we truly are.

Healers who today use traditional healing arts often incorporate a wide variety of therapies, including diet, herbs, acupuncture, and the laying on of hands, to strengthen the physical body and the life force within the individual. In my own work as a nurse practitioner, I use many healing modalities, often blending modern medical science with traditional healing practices. Over many years of practice, I have used healing touch extensively, relying on its remarkable powers to restore body, mind, and spirit to good health. This book is an outgrowth of my practice and strives to strike a balance between the often necessary use of medical treatments and ancient or traditional healing.

In this book, I'll talk about what scientific research has to say about the ancient practice of healing touch, but for the most part I'll be approaching the subject with the same understanding, respect, and spirit that traditional healers have applied since the birth of civilization. No other explanation better articulates how the practice actually works, and no other set of attitudes better prepares you to apply its principles.

The practice goes by many names. Dolores Krieger, Ph.D., R.N., a scientist and nurse and one of the pioneers of healing touch, and practitioner Dora Kunz have coined the term "therapeutic touch." Some refer to it as "a healing," and still others call the practice "healing through the auric field." Usually, I refer to the practice as healing touch, though all of these terms are essentially interchangeable. The reason is that whatever terms we use, the underlying principles are the same. Simply put, the practitioner of healing touch serves as a conduit, or channel, for a powerful healing energy that flows through the practitioner to the person he or she wishes to help.

Today, the practice of healing touch is being restored to a place of respect, thanks largely to the many medical, scientific, and lay practitioners who are using healing touch to help people overcome every sort of illness and problem.

This book will teach you how to use healing touch. It will show you how to make use of an energy that, at this moment, is flowing through your entire being. To the extent that it is possible, I will explain how therapeutic touch works and why it works. The book is intended for those of you who want to rediscover the healing power in your hands and utilize that power at whatever level you wish. You can apply healing touch to help yourself, your friends, and your loved ones. Or, with practice, study, and continual self-refinement, you can become a practitioner of this powerful healing tool.

As with most of the healing arts, healing touch makes its greatest demands of the practitioner. Throughout this book, I will be challenging many commonly held ideas and assumptions. I will be asking you to appreciate, at a much deeper level, the perceptions and abilities that arise from your senses, especially those that reside in your touch, and your intuition.

The Undiscovered Power of Touch

To greater and lesser degrees, all of us take our senses for granted, but perhaps no sense is more overlooked than our capacity for touch. Ironically, touch offers us a ceaseless and staggering amount of information every instant of our lives. Consider for a minute that right now your hands are providing you information about the book you are holding—the thickness of its pages and the sharpness of their edges, the resistance offered by the book's binding, the book's weight, and the slickness of its cover. If you are sitting, the nerves in your buttocks and legs are sending signals to your brain regarding the design and relative comfort of your chair. The temperature around you is conveyed by the air touching your skin. Your skin is also providing you information about the clothes you are wearing and the press of your feet against the floor. Touch provides you with a sense of place—not only with the gross matter that you touch but also with the warmth of the sun on your skin, or the push of the wind in your face, or the textured resistance of the soil beneath your feet. It tells us the temperature of water, the softness or coarseness of a person's skin, and the fine details of every surface we encounter. Without the ongoing sense of touch, you would be completely "out of touch" with the physical universe.

Each of us is introduced to physical life through the touch of our parents, the first and most essential way in which a mother and father communicate love to a child. Touch is also a fundamental means of communication between people.

On some level, all of us recognize that touch can convey healing power, especially if it is expressed with love. It is this very awareness that makes a parent want to rub or kiss a child's bruise, or hug a child who is emotionally or physically hurt. Indeed, loving touch is essential to our development. If a child is not given enough loving touch, the endocrine system will be impaired and the child will not grow properly. At the University of Miami Medical School, researchers found that premature babies experienced a 50 percent increase in weight gain when they received three fifteen-minute sessions per day of touching. The babies who received the touching were calmer, more active, and required fewer days in intensive care than those who did not receive the additional touching. Children who are abandoned and remain untouched frequently suffer from what medical doctors refer to as "failure to thrive." In fact, many elderly people who live alone and do not experience regular touching also develop this same syndrome.

The need to be touched continues through our lives. A hug, a kiss, lovemaking, and a rewarding pat on the back or shoulder—all of these are examples of how touch is used every day to communicate love, support, reconciliation, and even healing.

Somehow, we are able to discern a person's attitude and nature in his or her touch. Something almost tangible and full of information passes between us when we shake hands, touch someone on the shoulder, or hug someone. Indeed, our ability to receive information through touch is so refined that blindfolded parents are able to identify their newborn babies amid dozens of other infants merely by touching the children. By actively making such information conscious, we begin to open up to our incredible capacities of perception. We begin to open up to a larger definition of life that encompasses tangible and intangible connections to others.

Healing touch requires an even greater degree of sensitivity than touch or massage therapies, because the practitioner does not physically touch the recipient but passes his or her hands just over the person's body. As I will describe in detail later on, I sometimes touch the physical body to help move blocked or stagnant energy. For the most part, however, I perform the bulk of the treatment on the field itself, which is to say, slightly away from the actual physical body. The practitioner is seeking to heal and strengthen what traditional healers call the "life force," a complex web of energy that surrounds and permeates the human body.

Our culture has little understanding of how a person can influence the health of another human being without physically touching him or her. Our current worldview, which is based on the scientific objective model, insists that the world is made up of separate objects that have no relationship with each other unless they physically interact. This way of seeing life prevents us from understanding the subtle but powerful forces that link us all. It also prevents us from seeing how the practitioner of healing touch can act as a conduit for a powerful healing force that can be transferred from one person to another.

To better understand the process, let us first turn to the language and philosophy of our ancestors, and then see how modern science, in spite of its preconceptions and prejudices against ideas such as the "life force" and "human energy field," is validating this philosophy in the laboratory.

Beneath the Flesh and Bones, a Living Energy

Every traditional culture, whether it be Chinese, Japanese, Asian Indian, Greek, or Native American, sees life as an entity unto itself—a life force—that resides in physical objects for a certain amount of time. This life force is actually a vast and limitless energy, much like a river without beginning or end. That flow of life energy manifests as individual people, animals, insects, plants, and inanimate objects, such as rocks. The ancient Chinese called this infinite life force *chi;* the Greeks called it *pneuma;* the Asian Indians *prana;* the Japanese *Qi,* and Native Americans just referred to it as the Flow of Spirit.

Whatever the name, the flowing of a universal life force from the creator of the universe to each living thing is seen as the basis of physical, psychological, and spiritual health in virtually every traditional culture. Your body is infused with this life force. It surrounds and permeates every cell, organ, and sense. It is like a great ball of energy within which your body resides. As long as the life force flows through the human body, all the organs, systems, and senses function optimally. Illness is caused by a diminution in the flow of the life force. Without a free flow of life energy, organs function at lower rates of efficiency. Blood and lymph flows stagnate, waste accumulates, and illnesses manifest themselves.

No matter what therapies a traditional healer depends upon, he or she essentially is treating the life force itself. Wherever the life force is weak or deficient, the traditional healer attempts to make it strong; where it is too strong or excessive, the healer attempts to balance or modulate it. Restored to its optimal flow, the life force will assist the body's natural healing functions to restore health.

According to the traditional way of thinking, a person's way of life affects the degree to which he or she absorbs the life force, and thus enriches or impoverishes his or her existence. Practices that strengthen the life force within the individual eventually formed the basis for religious and spiritual life. For this reason, virtually every religious tradition depicts its spiritual teachers as having a glowing countenance. Evidence of the powerful life force emanating from spiritual figures abounds: In Buddhism, the Buddha radiates a golden glow; in Christianity, Jesus is shown with a glowing halo around his head. In the Bible and other religious books, these figures control the flow of that life force to bring healing to others (see, for instance, Mark 5:28–34).

Archaeologists have discovered in the Dead Sea Scrolls that the Essenes formally trained people in the laying on of hands, and that certain people within the Essene community possessed a marked ability to perform healing touch. Cave paintings of healing practices done by Native Americans depict the laying on of hands. Healing touch has been used throughout Asia. In fact, all Taoist philosophy, acupuncture, and the martial arts are based on developing a mature understanding and utilization of this underlying life force for health, wisdom, and personal power.

Growing Scientific Support

Today, scientists are validating this ancient wisdom. When researchers examine the effects of healing touch in the laboratory, they report consistent and even remarkable results.

At McGill University, in Montreal, Canada, Dr. Bernard Grad found that the wounds of laboratory mice that received healing touch healed faster than similar wounds on mice that did not receive therapeutic touch. Dr. Grad also found that plants that received therapeutic touch grew faster and stronger, and produced more chlorophyll, than plants that did not receive such treatment. Dr. Krieger reported that hemoglobin—the oxygen-carrying substance in human blood—increased in patients receiving therapeutic touch. Since hemoglobin is essential to life and healing, this suggested that therapeutic touch enhanced the body's capacity to heal itself. Other studies have supported such conclusions. Daniel Wirth, at the John F. Kennedy University Graduate School for Professional Psychology in Orinda, California, demonstrated increased wound healing in twenty-two of forty-four male student volunteers who were given five minutes of therapeutic touch treatments after having surgical incisions.

In 1987, Dr. Janet Quinn reported a significant improvement in immune function among subjects receiving therapeutic touch. Among her findings was an enhanced ratio between CD4 cells—the helper T cells that direct the immune response against an antigen—and CD8 cells—the cells that shut off the immune system. (The enhanced ratio of CD4 and CD8 cells is particularly important for people with HIV and AIDS. These people typically suffer from a diminishing number of CD4 cells and a stabilizing or increase in the number of CD8 cells. The drop in CD4 cells causes the immune system to rapidly decline, while the increase in CD8 cells causes the system to shut off, or to simply fail to respond in the presence of a pathogen or cancer cell.)

Studies have shown that those people receiving healing touch have increased alpha brain waves, characteristic of people in a meditative state. Such deep states of relaxation are associated with diminution of stress, improved respiration, better hormonal balance, enhanced bowel function, lower blood cholesterol levels, and heightened immune response. It's important to note that healing touch works on plants, animals, and humans (both in infants and adults), a fact that weakens the argument that the whole phenomenon is caused by a placebo effect. Also, there are no harmful side effects to such treatment. Healing touch is safe and highly effective. These and other studies reveal that something more than nerve fibers is involved in the exchange between the practitioner and recipient.

Developing a Scientific Model for the Energy Field

Not only are researchers demonstrating in the laboratory that healing touch works, they are also finding evidence for the underlying mechanisms that may explain *why* it works. Scientists are proving in the laboratory that the human body is animated by a complex web of electrical energy and that this underlying energy can be enhanced to bring about healing.

Among the leaders in this field of research is Robert Becker,

M.D., an orthopedic surgeon and formerly professor at Upstate Medical Center, Syracuse, N.Y. Dr. Becker and his colleagues have shown that a variety of techniques can boost the body's underlying electrical currents, which in turn strengthens the body's healing mechanisms, including the immune, endocrine, and nervous systems. Among the techniques Dr. Becker has shown to be effective at strengthening the body's energy system are acupuncture, certain dietary practices, and healing touch.

In his book *Cross Currents: The Perils of Electropollution; the Promise of Electromedicine* (Jeremy P. Tarcher, 1990), Dr. Becker reports that laboratory evidence is providing a picture of how healing touch may work.

"I have seen remarkable results obtained in a number of life-threatening circumstances," writes Dr. Becker. ". . . Since we know that the body uses electrical control systems to regulate many basic functions and that the flow of these electrical currents produces externally measurable magnetic fields, it does not require a great leap of faith to postulate that the healer's gift is an ability to use his or her own electrical control systems to produce external electromagnetic energy fields that interact with those of the patient. The interaction could be one of those that 'restores' balance in the internal forces or that reinforces the electrical systems so that the body returns toward a normal condition."

Dr. Becker and others have shown that by boosting the body's underlying electrical currents, the immune system and vital organs are also strengthened. Researchers have also demonstrated that the very act of healing is electrical in nature. That is, when the body is injured or ill, it struggles to increase the electrical energy flowing to the site of the injury or illness. This research forms the basis of a potentially revolutionary form of health care that scientists are calling "electromedicine." It has the potential to link modern science with ancient healing practices to create a truly unified medical system.

The basis for such healing, Dr. Becker has demonstrated, is the electrical body that surrounds and permeates the physical body.

Dr. Becker has shown that this energetic body, which he calls (as does Rupert Sheldrake, author of *A New Science of Life* and *The Rebirth of Nature*), a "morphogenic field," contains a unique intelligence that controls the growth, development, and health of cells and tissues.

As he describes in *Cross Currents,* Dr. Becker came by this discovery after performing a series of remarkable experiments on salamanders. These animals, you will recall, have the ability to regrow in perfect detail a new leg, an eye, an ear, half a heart, as much as one third of a brain, and most of a digestive tract.

The researchers at SUNY severed the tail and leg of a salamander, and as the animal grew new cells at the places of the amputations, Dr. Becker took some of the growing cells that were developing into a new tail and placed them on the stump of the amputated leg. You would think that these "tail cells" would continue to grow into a tail because DNA had already programmed them to do so. Remarkably, the new tail cells that were placed on the stump of the amputated leg became a new leg. The leg was complete in every detail, including skeletal bone, muscle, and nerves—all in perfect order!

On another salamander, Becker reversed the process: He took cells that were being used to grow a leg and placed them at the site of the amputated tail, and they grew into a perfectly developed tail. Becker was able to show that new cells, taken from any amputation site on the salamander's body and placed elsewhere at a new site, will become that new part of the body, whether heart, brain, or intestine. The question, of course, is: What made these cells become a leg, a complex organ by any standard, after they had already begun to grow into a tail? What changed the orders of the DNA?

The researchers were able to refute the notion that this change occurred locally, that is, at the site of the amputation by orders conveyed through local nerves. In fact, the researchers demonstrated that the nerves were "completely silent," which is to say, they transmitted no nerve impulses and no information. According to the reductionist view, the new-growing cells that were coded to grow a tail should have produced a tail—unless there was some larger intelligence that understood the salamander's body as a whole. This larger intelligence, which contains a blueprint of the animal's body, recognized the need to grow a new leg, and reordered the tail cells to produce a leg.

Through a series of additional experiments, Becker discovered that there was indeed a larger intelligence that existed as an electrical field that surrounds and infuses the salamander's body. Becker proved that this larger electrical body, a "morphogenic field," actually organizes and orders the DNA to produce whatever the body needs at a particular site. He proved that the information is passed from this morphogenic field to the animal's body, which triggers the appropriate DNA response and in turn produces the appropriate organ.

The morphogenic field also plays a role in the healing powers of acupuncture and healing touch. The field directs more life energy to specific parts of the body that need healing. Becker demonstrated that whenever a person is cut, injured, or suffers from an illness, the body increases the flow of direct-current electricity, which provides the essential energy for healing, to the injured or diseased site.

Acupuncture and therapeutic touch, to name just two forms of therapy, actually facilitate the focusing of additional energy to wounds and parts of the body that are diseased. Practitioners of healing touch perform this function by acting as conduits of life energy, which passes from the universal source, through the practitioner, and on to the recipient. In other words, the practitioner of healing touch performs the same function that the body itself is attempting to perform. The big difference is that, very often, the practitioner is able to boost the energy, which helps to overcome blockages to the life force and, in many cases, speeds the healing process.

Anyone Can Use Healing Touch

You can use healing touch to help a friend or family member who may be struggling with a chronic or acute disease or disharmony. With continued exposure to healing touch, you may also want to become a practitioner of this powerful healing tool. Those who have no intention of becoming a professional practitioner, however, must make a commitment to following all the steps in the practice, especially centering (see chapter 6). Working with someone who is ill can be extremely debilitating unless you are centered and know your limits. You also should be aware of the kinds of imbalances you will be treating and how to address these disharmonies. Specifically, you should know how to pull energy away from the field and direct it toward the individual. Finally, no session should be longer than thirty minutes, especially if you are new to the practice. Chapters 2, 3, 7, 8, and 10 provide instruction for time of treatment, sending and pulling energy, assessing the field, and using healing touch for specific imbalances. Read these chapters carefully before you employ the practice.

Joining the Modern with the Ancient for a Truly Holistic Healing Model

Scientists are on the threshold of learning a great deal about the electrical field, or energy body, that surrounds and infuses the physical form. But they have just scratched the surface. In order to have a working picture of this field, we must rely on the model given us by traditional healers and religious and spiritual teachers. This teaching, which I use in my own practice, has not been proven by science and likely never will be until we have scientific equipment with the sensitivity to measure this very subtle energy. Even if science could analyze this energy, it could not measure the ineffable qualities of the field, as it is understood by traditional people. That understanding extends too far into the realm of spirit to be comprehended by the current scientific method. Nevertheless, we need a picture of the energy body, which this model provides, to understand and perform this work. As you perform healing touch, you will develop your own experiences and understanding. For many of you, the model itself may change. You'll develop your own images of the character and topography of the energy body. But for now, let's see the practice in action and then explore the ideas and models that have served healers for more than ten thousand years.

2

✣

The Healing
Process

Wendy, a young woman on the verge of being crippled by multiple sclerosis, was twenty-eight when she first came to see me. Just before her first appointment with me in the spring of 1992, her doctor had informed her that her disease was worsening and that she should purchase a wheelchair immediately. In all likelihood, he said, she would be restricted to it by Thanksgiving. He also warned her to spend a week in the hospital to receive intravenous treatments of prednisone, a corticosteroid drug that suppresses the immune system and reduces inflammation. Prednisone has many side effects, however, including the weakening of bones and the encouragement of osteoporosis. Wendy wanted to try some other form of therapy first and eventually found her way to me.

I began by performing weekly treatments of healing touch and putting her on a program of dietary supplements. Before I recommend such supplements to any of my patients, I take a thorough medical history and advise them to get a thorough physical examination by their medical doctor if they have not already. I then do a complete blood analysis, from which I usually suggest dietary changes along with taking additional dietary supplements. These food supplements are prescription items in the wholistic field. They can only be dispensed by licensed health-care professionals. In Wendy's case, I suggested a program to clean her liver and support her digestion and nervous system.

At the time, Wendy suffered from many of the standard symptoms of MS, including the shaking of her limbs, stammer, weakness in the legs, shuffling of the feet, chronic fatigue, and a tendency to drop objects that she held in her hands. Her condition was complicated by asthma and sinusitis, which frequently caused labored breathing and wheezing. The muscles in her neck and shoulders were exceedingly stiff and hard. Conversely, her arms were weak and flaccid. In addition, the third and fourth fingers of her right hand were bent rigidly into the palm and could not be moved. In general, her fingers were numb and tingly, but the third and fourth fingers of the right hand had no feeling in them whatsoever.

Immediately, I realized that an excessive amount of Wendy's life force was bound up and blocked in her shoulders. These blockages prevented the life energy from moving down into her arms, hands, and legs, causing her limbs to get progressively weaker and, in the case of her fingers, progressively number. In order to help Wendy, I would have to free the energy that was locked in her shoulders and back and move it down into her arms and the lower parts of her body.

In a very deliberate manner, I began by removing the blocks to her energy and making it flow more freely throughout her field. This involved a kind of slow and gentle scooping action over her upper back. Whenever I pulled away the blocked, excessive energy from her back, I would literally send it up into the air. I asked Wendy to visualize the energy from her heart moving up into her throat, down each arm, and into her fingers, tendons, and bones. I then turned my attention to her arms, hands, fingers, and legs, and sent new energy into these tissues, tendons, and bones. As I worked on Wendy, my hands became very hot, an indication of the intense energy and circulation that was emanating from them, as well as the energy I was taking off her shoulders and neck.

After treating Wendy for a few weeks, an image came to my mind during one of our sessions. I saw a little girl sitting on a large black box with her thumb in her mouth. It was clear from the image that the little girl wouldn't open the box to explore it—but couldn't get off the box and leave it, either. She seemed stuck.

This image jumped into my mind with such clarity and force that I knew it had to be some kind of key to my treatment of Wendy. Very gently, and without any pretense that I "knew" something about her, I shared the image with Wendy and asked if it meant anything to her. Remarkably, the image of a little girl sitting on a black box had come to her as well. It seemed that as I worked on her, the image had passed from her field to mine, at which point I was able to make it conscious. At each subsequent session, Wendy and I engaged in the process of discovering what this image might mean to her and her healing. We explored many emotional issues that might lie within that black box. After each of these discussions, I would perform healing touch on Wendy.

We concluded that the black box symbolized Wendy's unconscious and that it held repressed emotions. The little girl indicated that Wendy had been emotionally traumatized at some early stage in life. Inside of the adult Wendy was a little girl who was suffering emotionally but was unable to deal with all the pain that was locked inside of her psyche. That pain had prevented the little girl from moving on and developing more fully. It manifested in the adult by preventing her from feeling physically when she was confronted with highly charged emotional situations. Hence, certain aspects of Wendy's consciousness were stuck in some preadolescent stage of development. These repressed and unexamined emotions within her psyche were stored in the black box upon which the little girl in the image sat. We also realized that those emotions, and the events that had triggered them, contained information and experiences that had to be examined and integrated into conscious life by the adult Wendy if she were to be healed.

In addition, I concluded that the energy that was stuck in her shoulders had originated in her heart chakra. Once it became blocked in her shoulders, it was unable fully to infuse her lungs, neck, arms, and hands.

Wendy characterized her emotional life as "going numb." She then suggested that perhaps her whole disease process was analogous to the way that she had gone numb emotionally.

I agreed, but only partially. I told Wendy that no one is to blame for his or her disease. On the contrary, no one fully understands all the reasons why he or she becomes ill. I stressed that in order for Wendy and me to work effectively, we must recognize that health and illness are mysteries that cannot be fully solved, but to which we must surrender.

Healing Is Transformative

This is an important concept to maintain as you read this book. The mind convinces us that we must *intellectually* understand the healing process in order to be healed, but that is merely the mind's attempt at maintaining control of the process itself—a veritable impossibility. True healing, especially from a serious disease, almost always involves personal transformation. Such healing includes confronting and changing deeply ingrained habits that have long been used to cope with life. This can be difficult since, very often, the habit was developed to help the person deal with emotional or psychological pain and survive it. Such habits once served an important purpose but now are no longer appropriate to the current situation or stage of life. By changing old ways of behaving, we renew ourselves and our lives. Thus we move into the future with new attitudes and more revitalizing ways of dealing with life— the past, present, and future. Since all of us maintain habits to cope with life, we are all growing and shedding behaviors at various stages of our development. No one, therefore, can be fully to blame for his or her illness, any more than healthy people can take full credit for being physically well.

Nevertheless, Wendy's own analysis of the numbness she experienced in her emotional life and in her physical body could be used as a therapeutic tool. "To feel is to heal," I suggested. "Perhaps this is some kind of guidance or mantra that you can use to encourage your recovery."

The energy work was having a very beneficial effect on Wendy. Increasingly, she felt strong enough to explore her emotional pain, to open the black box and examine its contents. At the same time, she was making excellent progress physically. In general, multiple sclerosis is marked by steady degeneration of the nervous system and the life-sustaining organs. The disease process is punctuated by plateaus that represent temporary periods of physical stability but that give way to another round of further degeneration of the nervous system and the organs it supplies. MS tends to worsen until any one of a number of life-threatening conditions that can eventually snuff out a person's life sets in. For this reason, MS is considered "incurable."

Contrary to all that was expected, Wendy was not experiencing the same type of steady decline. For one thing, she was walking regularly, and her gait was not weakening. In fact, we were working so well together that we were becoming hopeful that the work could slow the degenerative process somewhat and perhaps significantly improve her condition.

Entering the Healing Triangle

Wendy and I had entered what I refer to as the "healing triangle," an enhanced state of mind and body composed of three characteristics: patience, intention, and imagination (see diagram 1). As I continue to do this work, I am convinced that there is no disharmony on this planet that we cannot overcome. Yet, we need certain characteristics if we are to prevail and restore harmony to our lives. The first characteristic needed is patience, which contains within itself perseverance, humility, and concentration. According to *The American Heritage Dictionary,* patience is "the capacity of calm

DIAGRAM 1. THE HEALING TRIANGLE

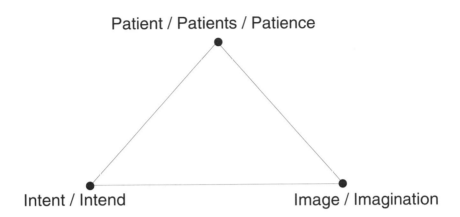

endurance." Patience gives us the strength to stay focused on our goal, to remain calm, and to endure in right action. Patience allows us to perform every task calmly and thoroughly so that the accumulation of these actions leads inevitably to our goal. Wendy demonstrated patience by allowing the healing process to unfold naturally and organically. If she was tired, she rested. If she didn't rest, she developed numbness in several parts of her body. As she honored her healing process and allowed it to progress at its own pace, her body became stronger and her bouts of fatigue and numbness became shorter.

Implicit within patience are humility and openness. Neither Wendy nor I had an agenda or schedule as to when she would begin to improve, or even what form the improvement would take. Rather, we were open to whatever her body decided to do with the energy being channeled through me to her. We knew we were seeing significant signs of improvement when she was able to distinguish by feel what kind of coin she was holding in her hand while her eyes were closed. She also became able to attend exercise class regularly and do all of the exercises. As Wendy improved, her gait was more stable and she no longer had numbness in her legs and feet. However, if she became overtired and did not rest properly, her gait would lag and the numbness return. Overall, we were en-

couraged by her progress and felt a renewed sense of patience and
faith in her healing process.

The second point on the triangle that Wendy and I utilized is
intention. Again, the dictionary tells us that to intend is to have a
"clear purpose; an aim that guides action . . ." Such characteristics
imply a strong will—the willpower to move toward a goal in the
face of doubt. At the outset of the relationship between the healer
and recipient, the healer is usually the one with the clearest intention and the strongest belief in what she or he is doing. The recipient may come to you simply because, as in Wendy's case, you are
the only alternative to a wheelchair and prednisone treatments. Yet,
the recipient may be filled with doubts. He or she may not have any
belief that the practice can be of benefit. In this case, the patient
needs strong intention toward his or her goal and the honesty and
the willingness to objectively assess the effects of the practice.
Meanwhile, the healer must also have strong intention and the will
to move forward in the face of her own doubts. Oh, yes, even the
healer must deal with doubts: Can this person get well? Can the
practice help him or her? Can I perform the practice adequately so
that this person benefits? These are just a few of the doubts that
creep into the heart of every healer who truly wants to help others.
To move beyond such doubts, the healer, too, needs clear intention.

With time and her physical improvement, Wendy began to
believe in healing touch, as well. Once she saw the results, Wendy
and I were working together with strong patience and intention.

Finally, patience and intention combine to create a higher possibility, which exists initially in the world of image and imagination, the third leg of the healing triangle. Imagination that arises out
of the practice of patience and intention creates possibilities that
were not initially apparent, nor originally seen or even dreamed of.

The healing path described by the characteristics that com-
prise the healing triangle is a very different path from that traveled
by those who are ill and act out of fear. Some people who act exclusively from fear have little patience and no clear intention (except to escape the illness). Trying to rush the healing process toward

a preconceived goal obscures one's ability to see the possibilities for creating wellness that may be implicit in the situation. On the other hand, by maintaining patience and acting with clear intent, we invite the magic of healing because we are open to the third element in the alchemical mix: imagination.

Many adults believe imagination to be something that resides mostly in children, something one grows out of. We're taught to grow into realism. Be realistic, we are told. We even shame one another by telling our friends to be realistic. It's like saying "Grow up" or "Act your age."

This "adult" way of thinking limits our creativity and, in the process, limits the possibilities for our healing. Fortunately for all of us, imagination cannot be killed or completely wiped out of our faculties, for it is a fundamental part of our humanness. It fuels our creativity. So, although we have unspoken rules about how we can apply our imagination, and while we are selective in how we use it, we can relearn how to gain access to it.

Using our imagination to aid the healing process is not a modern practice. Traditional peoples around the world always have been highly imaginative in their ways of healing, and are just as effective in treating many kinds of illnesses and disorders. Healing touch and other forms of energy medicine, such as herbs and nutrition, have been healing people since the dawn of consciousness. Today, science is recanting its condemnation of these practices, yet in us there is still that subtle training that works against our rightful claim to these and other forms of healing and also prevents us from using our imagination to conjure images of health and wellness.

Bad health, on the other hand, you can be imaginative about. Bad health, you can predict; you can even be clairvoyant when it comes to predicting your own bad health. "I think I'm about to be sick" is a perfectly legitimate thing to say. But people look askance at those who are already ill but say "I feel very strongly that I'm about to get well." We tend to offer a patronizing smile to the person who says words like that. Many people—especially health professionals—are threatened when people talk imaginatively about their imminent good health. The reason for this is that people tend to trust their assessment of bad symptoms, such as nausea or headache, but the prediction that you're going to get better because you're experiencing positive symptoms is often categorized as wishful thinking or "unrealistic" optimism.

Imagination is the gateway to seeing yourself and your world in larger, unrestricted terms. Imagination is also the basis for the positive messages that you send to your cells, organs, and overall body: "I am healthy" is a very positive message to your cells. It can even program them to act in ways that promote health. Imagination is the mother lode that you can tap into—like a big vein of gold in a dark mine—that can yield all kinds of rich and even magical possibilities. The third element in the healing triangle, imagination, points the way upward to good health. Imagination is an essential ingredient in every recovery, no matter what type of therapy is utilized.

We must remember, however, that what we imagine may be smaller than what can be achieved or is intended by the Creator. Our imagination has been put down for so long that we must acknowledge that perhaps greater possibilities exist than even those we can imagine. Think of imagination as the opening of your arms. It is the reaching up and welcoming the possibility of the unexpected, even the magic, that life provides for rebirth.

The Triangle Becomes a Pyramid

The triangle, of course, is a two-dimensional object, an abstract design that has height and width but no depth. When traditional people utilized the triangle to create spiritual temples, shrines, and symbols for healing, they gave the triangle a square base by adding two points, one in the front and another in the back, thus creating a pyramid. To carry our triangle metaphor one step further, therefore, I want to add two more points to the triangle's base to create a healing pyramid. These two points are gratitude and faith, two virtues that are so intimately related that each one gives rise to the other (see diagram 2).

Gratitude, as the pioneer stress researcher Hans Selye pointed out, has the power to instantaneously change your entire attitude toward life. Once you look at your life with gratitude, everything around you suddenly has an extremely important value. You notice the beauty of nature, the smiles of your loved ones, the goodness in your friends, and the endless blessings that you have received in life. You recognize that at so many vitally important junctures in life, situations whose outcomes were extremely tenuous nevertheless turned in your favor. One can hardly experience gratitude and feel the weight of its many revelations without wondering about the source of it all and the ultimate benevolence of that source. Like Plato and Socrates, we are forced to wonder if there isn't some force

DIAGRAM 2. THE HEALING PYRAMID

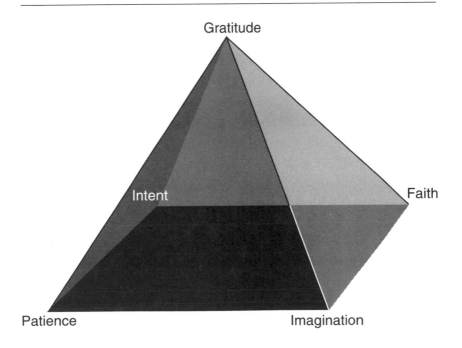

for good behind life's events. The more we consider that source, the more we come to have faith in it. Thus, gratitude leads inevitably to faith.

As Wendy and I worked together, she began to talk about how much she had learned from healing touch, and even from her illness. She had learned how to honor and respect her body, to rest it when it needed rest, and to nourish it with better-quality food and drink. The more intimate she became with her body, the more she marveled at its endless mysteries. That intimacy and wonder gave her even more gratitude for her body and greater faith in the ever-unfolding healing process.

I could not help but be grateful that Wendy had come into my life. I had learned so much from working with her and had gained so much more confidence in my abilities and in the efficacy of the practice. These were irreplaceable gifts she had given me, gifts that had changed my life.

Healing Is a Gift You Give Yourself

One day in June, while working on Wendy, I felt overcome by a strange calm sensation, a feeling of tremendous well-being. I was moving the energy out of Wendy's back and neck, down her arms, and into her hands. I then turned my attention to her hands, especially her right hand, where the third and fourth fingers were bent inward with almost a spastic quality. I was very focused and aware only of her hand and curled fingers. Suddenly, I was moved to hold her hand and her third and fourth fingers, and then, very gently, I straightened them. Wendy's hand opened and her fingers stretched out to their full length. Slowly and cautiously, she began to flex her fingers, moving them back and forth. These fingers had been rigid and immovable for months and now they were straight. For a moment, I couldn't believe what I had just witnessed and participated in. I looked at Wendy in disbelief. "You opened your hand," I said.

As if she were reading my mind, Wendy said, "Yes, Deby,

you really opened my hands." She started to cry. At that moment, I felt that God was moving through me. I wasn't questioning anymore.

From that time onward, Wendy made tremendous progress in her healing. I worked on her regularly for the next three years. Her legs got stronger, and she was able to stay on her feet and walk for longer distances before she became tired. She never needed a wheelchair, nor did she undergo prednisone treatments. Her hands and sensory perception continued to get stronger. Today, Wendy is the active mother of three children. She has completed a course that qualifies her as a nurse's aide, and now has a rewarding career and a family life that express the free-flowing energy of her heart. She has regained not only the ability to use her hands without artificial assistance but also her sensitivity to the size, shape, and texture of objects, which she can now identify with her hands. She can pick up coins and actually feel them. The tingling in her fingers is significantly reduced. Her nails are pink, an indication that the circulation in her fingertips is greatly improved. Whenever she overstresses herself, her legs get numb, but as long as she walks and exercises within her limits, she is quite functional.

I still see Wendy from time to time for energy work, but not on the regular basis that I did in the beginning of our work. Just before we stopped seeing each other regularly, another image of her jumped into my mind. I saw her walking through a forest toward a radiant sun that was pouring light through the trees directly in front of her. To her immediate left and right was darkness. I shared this image with her and the two of us talked about it at length. We decided that the light was the path of healing, but behaviors that did not support her healing were deviations from that path, a detour, left or right, into the darkness that is illness.

The healing pyramid teaches us that we must accept the energy that the practice of therapeutic touch provides if the larger possibilities of the healing process are to occur. We must enter into the healing pyramid, so to speak. We must cultivate patience, intention, and imagination. We must experience gratitude and through gratitude develop faith. This is our part in the drama that is healing. And because we have an essential part in the healing process, we must understand that healing is a gift we give ourselves. We strive for patience, we maintain clear intent, and we open our arms to the possibilities that we may not at first see; we are transformed by gratitude, which ultimately gives us the gift of faith.

EXERCISE

1. Use a dictionary and thesaurus and list each word from the healing pyramid and its various meanings on separate index cards.
2. Read each card before a healing session to begin to activate the healing triangle and healing pyramid.

3

Using Your Hands to Heal

Humans have built civilizations, created great works of art, and healed one another with their hands. So much of our advancement as a species is based on a simple yet singular belief: that what the mind envisions the hands can create. The hands are the instruments of the imagination, and if the imagination is inspired by God, then the hands are the tools of the divine. The hands are themselves great works of art. They possess beauty, power, and utility. In the hands, raw strength, miraculous precision, and musical dexterity become one. The hands can build bridges, sculpt stone, type, tie flies, and perform surgery. All the powers of our minds, hearts, and souls are concentrated in our hands, which is why they are capable of reshaping the world. Who can deny that the hands possess a unique and even awesome power?

That power flows from your hands, and you can use it to heal. All you need is to develop your understanding of this practice and your confidence in its efficacy, and open your heart with love and understanding so that the life force can flow through your hands freely.

The Body Electric: On the Brink of a Medical Revolution

When I talk about the hands as radiating electromagnetic energy, and about the electromagnetic field that surrounds the body, I am not talking about something mystical or even speculative. I am talking about a scientific fact. The body is an electrical unit, and like all electrical units it is surrounded by an electrical field. Electricity makes your heart beat, your muscles expand and contract, and your nervous system send messages across tiny fibers of tissue. Within your brain, electrical impulses fire across the neurons, making every thought, mood, and physical reaction that you experience possible. In short, there isn't a single event that takes place in your body that isn't dependent upon an electrical charge.

A little more than five decades ago, scientists began photographing this human electrical field. In 1939, a Russian scientist by the name of Semyon Kirlian accidentally shocked himself with a high-voltage generator and saw an electrical flash discharge from his hands. Amazed by the brilliant release of energy, Kirlian created a camera that could photograph the electrical discharge coming off his fingers. In these photographs, that discharge appears as a halo full of spikes around the perimeter of the hands. For the next twenty years, he and his wife worked together in an attempt to discover if the electrical discharge being given off by the hands could be used as a diagnostic tool. Is it possible, the Kirlians wondered, that photographic images could be used to determine health and illness? The Kirlians mapped out an extensive set of images that they said could be used to determine various disease states. Meanwhile, the images were so startling that many scientists argued that these pictures were photographic proof of the body's "aura," which traditional healers and mystics had been talking about for millennia. Others maintained that these images were nothing less than physical evidence of the soul.

Western scientists didn't know what to make of the Kirlians' photographs and dismissed them as meaningless—at least until recently. Today, scientists at the Massachusetts Institute of Technology, the State University of New York, and other research centers are studying the body's electromagnetic field to find out "what can be seen through the new window," in the words of MIT biomagnetic researcher David Cohen. One of the reasons for this breakthrough in interest is that some scientists now report that the "aura" given off by the body changes according to the person's inner state.

In the late 1970s, biophysicist Leonard W. Konikiewicz and his colleagues at the Polyclinic Medical Center in Harrisburg, Pennsylvania, showed that negative feelings, such as apprehension and animosity, weaken the intensity of the inner corona given off by the hands. Conversely, joy and sexual excitement make the corona stronger. Further research demonstrated that the corona changes according to the physical condition within the body, such as the stage of the menstrual cycle and the person's overall physical health. A person with cancer, for example, gives off a brighter and more diffuse corona than a person in normal health. Researchers of Kirlian photography have long maintained that a tight, bright corona is a sign of health, while a larger, more diffuse corona is a sign of disease.

American biochemist Glen Rein, who at the time of his research worked at Queen Charlotte's Hospital in London, used Kirlian photography to study tissue samples from women with breast cancer, and compared them with samples from healthy women. Rein found that the light intensity emitted from the tissues of the women with breast cancer was greater and larger than that from the tissues of healthy women. Rein went on to show that the hands of cancer patients also discharged more electromagnetic energy than those of people in good health. Some researchers speculate that the increase in energy released from cancer patients reveals that the body is in a state of degeneration, and consequently can no longer hold the life force in its grasp. Hence, the energy is released in greater quantities and shows up on Kirlian images as a larger, brighter, and more diffuse corona.

My own experience with cancer has given me a slightly different understanding of this phenomenon. The cancer cells, or tumor, are consuming the life force at such a rapid rate that they are responsible for this discharge of excess energy that is perceived in Kirlian photography. The life force was being drawn away from healthy cells and siphoned off to the cancer. This causes a general breakdown of the body, or the loss of physical and energetic integrity, which is revealed by Kirlian pictures as the excessive or unhealthy glow that radiates from the fingertips.

Other experiments have shown that the intensity of the corona also changes according to the environmental factors a person finds himself in. These factors include the temperature in the room the person is in, those who are present in the room with him, and the feelings of those present. In other words, the relative strength or weakness of the field depends a great deal upon both the inner and outer conditions of the person being examined. (This is one reason why I stress in chapter 6 how important centering is and how vital it is that you, the practitioner, be aware of your inner condition when you do this work.)

Scientists all over the world are now taking energy medicine to new vistas. Some of the work is far ahead of that being done in prestigious universities, such as MIT and SUNY, but it nevertheless describes where scientists may be looking in the years ahead. One such pioneer is Harry Oldfield, a London scientist who has developed a technique called "electronography." Oldfield's technique is to send a low-energy electromagnetic field through the body, which absorbs some of the field and radiates the rest back at a sensitive device that can detect a spectrum of frequencies being emitted from the body. Oldfield maintains that each organ has its own frequency, or vibratory rate, and that it can be detected and measured to determine the health of that organ. He has shown that when a person is thinking about something pleasant the body's electrical field is stronger. When a person thinks of something depressing or frightening, the field becomes significantly weaker.

Oldfield's work was reported in the spring 1986 issue of *Advances,* the prestigious journal of the Institute for the Advancement of Health. Writing about the technique, Clive Wood, Ph.D., a phys-iologist who teaches at Oxford University, experienced Oldfield's method firsthand. "Oldfield asked if he could scan my jaw and accurately located some recent dental bridgework that he could not have known about," wrote Wood. "Scanning my solar plexus, he asked me to think of something unpleasant. I thought about the dentistry, and within seconds the needle allegedly monitoring the energy output fell almost to zero. The thought, he said, had altered the relationship between the energy frequencies going into and coming out of my body. If it was a trick, it was a good one, but he had no reason to deceive me."

While Oldfield and others work on the outer rim of electro-magnetic medicine, many highly regarded scientists are demon-strating the more fundamental fact that the body is not only an electromagnetic unit but that it can direct energy to heal. As I pointed out in chapter 1, Robert Becker at SUNY showed that all healing involves an increase in the flow of electromagnetic energy to the impaired part of the body. Becker's and Oldfield's work, when looked at together, may explain how an increase in positive thinking results in a stronger immune response: Positive thoughts may trigger a stronger electrical field, which may in turn boost im-mune function. This research may also explain why such practices as biofeedback and positive imaging have such healing effects.

That the body is an electrical unit, and that health is depen-dent on electromagnetic energy, is now well established. You have the power not only to heal yourself by boosting your own electrical field but also to help others by boosting theirs. That power radiates from all parts of your electromagnetic field. You can use your hands to direct that power to others.

"Turning On" the Hands

Once you center yourself, the next step is to "turn on" your hands, meaning to get the energy flowing powerfully from your hands. To do that, you must become conscious of the life force flowing through you from a higher source, or the Universal Healer. That energy flows to you from the cosmos above and the earth below, the two poles of existence. It fills your field and your entire body and flows like a powerful current to your hands. Your hands have the power to direct this current of healing energy to your client.

In this chapter, we are going to perform several exercises so that you can experience the healing power that flows from your hands. We'll begin simply by focusing on the palms of your hands. Turn your palms upward and see if you can sense an energy resting in your palms, as if a very light ball were sitting in each of your hands. Many people can sense this energy right away, but don't be troubled if you cannot. It takes time to develop an awareness of energy as an entity unto itself—your own as well as another's. Now, let's explore that energy a little further.

First, rub your palms vigorously together for about one minute. With your fingers and palms flat and straight, hold your palms facing each other and keep them about eight inches apart. Now, slowly bring your palms toward each other. As you do, see if you can sense the energy being compressed between your palms, as if its density is offering your hands some resistance. Now, move your hands away from each other until they are about a foot apart. Note that it's slightly easier to move your hands away from each other than it is to move them toward each other. Do this a couple of times and gauge the relative resistance you feel as your hands go toward each other and away.

Again start out by vigorously rubbing your palms together for about one minute. This time, however, change the posture of your hands so that each hand is cupped, as if it were holding a ball. Gradually, move your hands toward each other in the same way you did earlier. Do not let them touch, but hold them about four inches apart. This time, see if you can sense a greater resistance between your hands than you could when your hands were flat. A cupped hand will sense energy easier than a flat palm will. You may also feel heat or a radiating type of energy between your palms. What you are feeling are characteristics of the energy itself.

If you are having difficulty feeling the energy in your hands by rubbing the palms together, try this exercise. Extend your hands directly out in front of you, at about shoulder height, with your palms facing upward. Quickly, open and close each hand thirty or forty times. Bring your hands together slowly in a cupped position and try to feel the energy between your hands. Many people perceive the energy between the hands as a spongy ball. The rapid squeezing of your hands awakens the secondary chakras located there.

Once you have established this sensitivity in your hands or "turned your hands on," ask a family member or friend to allow you to feel the energy around them. Your pets or plants also make good energy subjects. Do not touch the person but bring your hand within eighteen inches of his or her body. See if you can sense the density of the field. Move your hand a little closer and see if you can perceive the energy radiating from the body. If you can feel it, you will note that the field becomes firmer as your hand moves closer.

As you do these exercises, part of you will clearly sense the energy in your hands or radiating from another person's body. At the same time, another part of you will doubt your experience. It isn't your senses that are in conflict, but your competing definitions of what is real. As I said earlier, healing touch forces us to confront our current beliefs and definition of reality. In a way, I had an advantage over many people who begin this practice because I had already seen the power of touch to heal in my nursing practice. Each time I would stroke a person's hand, or touch an arm or a shoulder, I could feel my patients relax. It was as if the tension that had gripped their bodies was suddenly released.

Keep in mind that tension in the tissues of the body is the basis for many illnesses. Tension is nothing more than an increase of energy—and sometimes excessive energy—that has manifested in muscles and connective tissues, such as fascia.

Building the Spongy Energy Ball

Here is a meditation designed to increase awareness and the healing power in your hands; it will show you how to use that enhanced sensitivity to "feel" another person's energy field. First, become aware of the energy flowing to you from the Universal Healer, who sends it forth from the cosmos above and the earth below. See the energy fill your field and flow in great rivers of energy through your body. You are imbued with the power that the Great Healer is sending to you.

Now to expand the hand exercise from the previous page, rub your hands together vigorously until you can feel the warmth generated by the friction. Rubbing the hands together awakens the energy centers in the palms of your hands. Slowly allow your hands to separate until they are about twelve inches apart. Once they have reached that point, slowly bring your hands together, all the while feeling the energy compress between your hands. One of the first things you will notice in this exercise is that it is easier to separate your hands than to bring them together. It's as if something is pushing your hands apart. As you bring your hands toward one another, you can sense a certain resistance between your palms, as if the energy is being compressed and is thus getting denser. Whenever I do this exercise (and I do a form of it every time I work on a person's field) I am aware of a powerful ball of energy that now resides between my hands. I sense it as spongy and radiating light, about the size of a basketball (see diagram 3).

While maintaining that heightened sensitivity and awareness of the energy in your hands, walk up to a family member, a friend, or a coworker and gently bring your hand to within about eighteen inches of his or her shoulder or back. (Do not do this exercise without first asking the person's permission.) If the person is a spouse, your child, or a close and trusted friend, you may bring your hand a little closer. Do not touch the person, however. See if you can sense the density of the field around that person. Feel the energy radiating from his or her body. Later on, we'll define the field's

DIAGRAM 3. THE SPONGY ENERGY BALL

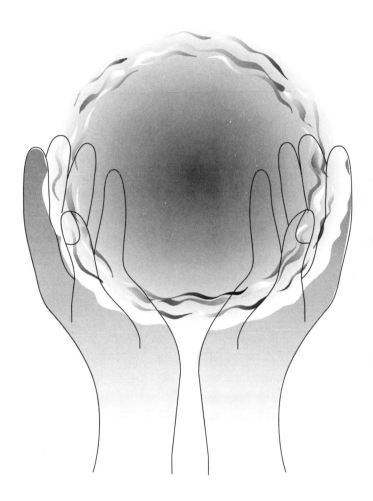

characteristics, but for now simply see if you can sense the energy that radiates from another person's body. If you can, you will note that the field is clearly palpable and even gets firmer as your hand moves closer to the body.

The more you become aware of your hands, the more you realize their remarkable power both to receive and to send energy. You can give energy to another person in the form of that ball of light that radiates from your palms. And you can receive energy—

and the information that is transmitted with it—when you shake hands or touch another person.

Relieving Pain: Jack's Story

Several years ago, I was providing nutrition counseling to a middle-aged man named Jack. Just after we began our work together, Jack suffered a heart attack and immediately underwent coronary by-pass surgery to restore blood and oxygen flow to his heart. At the time, surgeons were using part of the saphenous vein in the leg to replace the coronary arteries that supply the heart. One day after the surgery, he came into my office for our scheduled visit, and after we finished talking about his diet, I asked him if there were any other problems. Jack told me that his leg and ankle were both swollen and still very much in pain after the surgery. When I examined both, I saw that his ankle ballooned above the opening of his shoe, his foot was so swollen that he could barely put on his shoe, and his leg was inflamed and raw at the site of the incision. I offered to do healing touch on his leg. Jack balked. He didn't know anything about therapeutic touch and was skeptical. He preferred the more practical dietary recommendations I was giving him. "The practice can be effective against pain and swelling," I said. "It's worth a try."

"Let's do it, then," Jack said.

I asked Jack to remove his shoes and lie down on the table, where I began the treatment. I started by sending healing energy to the incision in Jack's leg. I then moved down to the ankle and removed the stagnant energy from the area of the swelling. I had expected only to be able to reduce Jack's pain, but as I continued to do the work, Jack's ankle felt less swollen to me but since his shoes were off, I couldn't judge the swelling adequately. However, I continued the treatment—removing stagnant energy from the ankle and sending the tissues healing life force. When I finished the treatment, Jack got up and tested his leg and found that the pain was gone. He walked around the room in amazement. "God, I can't believe this," he said. "I could never tell the doctor about this. He'd never believe it." He then put his shoes on, whereupon we both discovered that the swelling in his ankle had diminished noticeably. Both of us were now amazed. Jack walked around the room, shaking his head and saying, "This feels great. I can't believe it. I can't tell anyone about this. They'll think I'm crazy."

I continue to see Jack for nutritional counseling periodically. Although I do not provide energetic work for him, his wife, who later became my student, does.

Experiencing the Energy

This exercise will give you the experience of feeling the energy in your hands. It's a good exercise to perform before you work on someone's field.

EXERCISE

1. Hold your palms face up with arms slightly extended from your body.

2. Rapidly open and close both palms thirty to forty times.

3. Bring your slightly cupped hands slowly toward each other in front of you, noting the "spongy" ball of energy between your hands when they are about four inches apart.

Sending Energy and Pulling It from the Field

In my energy work with Wendy, I was essentially opening blocks and balancing the energy in her entire field. Her arms, hands, and legs were the areas that were deprived of energy, while her shoulders and back were burdened with blockages. I had to be able to remove energy where it was excessive and send it to places where it was deficient. It is not hard to determine where the energy is excessive or deficient, even before you become sensitive and experienced in being able to "feel" the energy with your touch. Remember that quality and quantity of energy within the field are generally replicated in the body itself. In Wendy's case, there was lots of blocked and excessive energy over her back and shoulders, which was manifested as rigid muscles in her neck and upper back. As for the field itself, I could palpably feel the energy when I moved my hands over and through this part of her field. It was dense and even heavy; it felt as if my hand were moving through a viscous substance that was full of resistance. Her arms, hands, and legs were deficient of energy, which was clearly reflected in the fact that these parts of her body were weak, and became more deficient when Wendy became overwhelmed with emotions of anger and fear. She would become immobilized—metaphorically speaking, she was unable to move off her black box and move along her healing path. Her fears prevented her from imagining her own good health and therefore prevented her from using the power of the healing triangle. When I worked on the field over these parts of her body, the lack of energy was palpable. The field felt distinctly empty, with no sense of charge, vitality, or density. This was a strange feeling for me as a practitioner of healing touch, because I had come to expect some reassuring sense of presence in the energy field.

My basic approach to Wendy's problem was to pull the energy out where it was blocked and excessive, and push the energy into the places where it was deficient. So, to help you get a feeling for working on pulling and pushing the energy, to help you experience the different sensations of therapeutic touch, try each of the following exercises.

You'll need a friend or partner to help you with this exercise.

EXERCISES

First, sit opposite each other in a straight-backed chair with your feet flat on the floor and your knees almost touching those of your friend. Take a minute or two to breathe deeply and center yourselves.

Now, rest your arms and hands on your thighs with your left palm facing upward and your right palm facing down. Have your partner place her right palm on top of your left palm and her left palm under your right palm. (For this exercise, you may actually touch each other's palms.)

Before you begin sending or receiving energy, you and your partner should try to determine how the energy is flowing between you. Does it go out your left hand and into your partner's right? Does the energy pass from your partner's right hand to your left? How does the energy that you receive from your partner affect your body? How does it travel through your body—that is, does it enter your right hand, for example, and travel up the arm, through the shoulders, and out the left hand? Try to feel the movement of energy before you try to affect the energy. Don't worry if you can't feel the flow of energy. Most important, don't think. Just feel. It takes time and practice to become sensitive to the movements of this energy.

Sending or Pushing the Energy to Your Partner

Once you have tried to establish the direction of the energy, see if you can direct it with your hands and mind. Decide between the two of you who is going to send the energy and who is going to receive it. Before you start to push the energy, take some deep breaths to center yourself. Decide which hand you are going to push the energy out of—the left or right. Now, use the exhalation of your breath to send the energy from the palm that you've chosen to send with. As you exhale, visualize the energy going out of your palm and into the opposite hand of your partner. The person who is receiving should stay in neutral mode and be sensitive to the energy. Visualize the line of flow—that is, see how the energy travels through your partner, such as from her arm, across her shoulders, down her other arm, returning to the hand opposite your own. Feel your other hand receive the energy. Ask your partner whether or not she can feel the energy flow. Take turns pushing with different hands. Also take turns receiving and sending the energy.

In general, sending energy to your partner or client will raise, or boost, the recipient's life energy. You send energy to places that are weak or deficient of Qi, or life force.

Pulling the Energy from Your Partner

The next energy flow to learn is pulling the energy. Pulling the energy will diminish the life force in an area; you do this in places where the energy is excessive. Repeat the previous exercise, but instead of pushing energy with the exhalation, visualize pulling the energy out of your partner's hand as you inhale. Try to determine how the energy is flowing within yourself and your partner. Where is the energy coming from that you are pulling from your partner? Is it coming from her shoulder? Her back? Her neck? Ask your partner if she has any physical sensations while you are pulling the energy from her.

Stopping the Energy Flow

Finally, let's try to stop the energy from flowing between you. Visualize the energy remaining at a state of rest between you and your partner. You are both closed to each other. Shut off. Determine how this feels and compare it to the previous exercises.

These exercises will help you learn how to master the ways in which you can direct energy through your hands. You can practice sending and receiving energy all day—whenever you shake a person's hand, send your energy or receive his or hers. When you touch another person on the shoulder or the arm, try to sense the person's energy or send some of your own. In short, try to expand your sense of touch. It's actually a lot easier than you think. Try not to make the practice excessively intellectual or difficult. All you need to do is experience and practice it.

Whenever you are sending or receiving energy, you will get images and impressions. As with the images I got when working with Wendy, these thoughts can help the healing process. At first, these impressions may be formless, but pay attention to the first thought that comes into your mind. It is usually correct. You may have a clear sensation that energy is moving out of your body to the recipient, yet your mind immediately attempts to squelch such a thought. You may hold your hand near a person's shoulder and immediately feel that you are able to sense the vibration coming from the person's field, yet your mind will automatically doubt what you are sensing. Learn to trust your initial perceptions and your expanded sense of touch.

In order to augment your practice, try to determine where the blockages exist in the people you see on the street or at work. Examine their fields and note the way they walk, or bend, or hold themselves. See if you can determine whether the left side or the right side of the field is stronger or weaker, whether there are blockages over the shoulders or neck or lower back. Try to "feel" the energy of a person you are sitting across from, and note any changes that take place in the person's field as you interact with this person.

With time and practice, all of these exercises become second nature. Your study of energy can go on all day long and for the rest of your life, with beneficial effects on your own and others' health.

Keep the Treatments Short

In general, healing touch sessions are short—anywhere from five to thirty minutes, depending on the age of the person and his or her health. The general rules are as follows: The younger the patient, the shorter the treatment time. And the more severe the disharmony of the person, the shorter the treatment.

For example, treatment for infants up to one year of age usually takes only thirty seconds. For a child of this age, you would do gentle healing touch over the area of disharmony or over the general body, especially in the case of premature babies or infants who are struggling with some type of systemic problem.

Ages one to five usually are treated for one minute (or for however long the child will sit still).

Very ill patients (especially those who are bedridden) are treated for no less than five minutes but no more than seven minutes. You can apply the treatment daily.

For those who suffer from acute illness (such as the first stage of a cold), the general rule is that less is more, meaning that a few minutes of healing touch will promote healing without overwhelming the body. If you work on a person with a cold or flu too long, you may trigger even stronger symptoms and more suffering than would otherwise have occurred. Colds are actually the body's attempt to eliminate accumulated waste and toxins, especially those that have been taken in from the environment, such as can be found in the air, water, and food. Over time, these waste products accumulate in the fluid between tissue cells. Tension in the muscles, fascia, and other tissues prevents the waste from moving into the lymph. Tension also prevents the lymph from moving the waste out of the tissues and into the liver for elimination. Hence, waste accumulates. This toxic environment in the tissues provides the right conditions for a virus or bacteria to flourish and to bring on a cold. Cold symptoms—such as sneezing, coughing, runny nose, frequent urination, diarrhea, and fever—are all the body's efforts to cleanse the system of toxins and to destroy the virus or bacteria. The symptoms are, in fact, the body's answer to the problem. By performing a long healing touch session on someone with a cold, you can trigger an even deeper discharge or elimination of waste products, and thus intensify the symptoms and cause more suffering. Thus, a cold or flu can be extremely acute in a twenty-four to forty-eight hour period. In other words, you will increase the suffering of the patient significantly. Treat this type of disharmony for five to seven minutes. You can apply the treatment daily. (For more on treatment of individual disorders, including the common cold, see chapter 10.)

One of the most difficult things to realize, especially when you are first starting out as a healing touch practitioner, is how powerful

DIAGRAM 4. TRANSFERRING OF ENERGY FROM THE ENERGY BALL TO THE SHOULDER

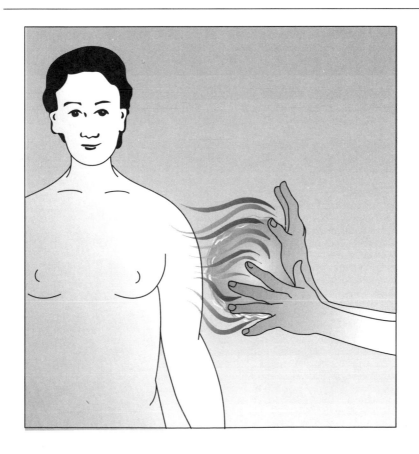

healing touch really is. You are sending another person the power of the life force, the basic energy that keeps the entire body alive (see diagram 4). Once the body accepts that energy, its own healing forces are boosted dramatically. What the body does with such energy and power is now up to that person and the Great Spirit.

Your hands have power. But as I intimated in the opening paragraphs of this chapter, that power flows from the mind and heart. And thus, your hands pour forth healing energy or fall inert by the images your mind and heart permit. You can limit your healing ability, or you can participate in a drama far greater than any of us can imagine. What mighty works these hands can perform, if only we have the faith to let them do their divinely inspired labor.

4

✻

The Energy Field

The vast majority of us can sense another person's energy field. In fact, very often the field is so palpable that most people perform mental and linguistic gymnastics in order to express in rational terms what we sense intuitively but cannot adequately explain. Thus, we refer to some people as having a "strong presence" or a "weak presence." We describe people who are thin or frail as having "a delicate energy." "He's a lightweight," someone says of another. "She fills up the room when she enters it." We don't really mean that a person is so wide that he or she "fills the room." We're talking about our clear perception of a person's energy field and all the information we derive from such perceptions.

Each of us senses the energy body and the consciousness that each energetic field contains. Some people radiate discipline, for example, or wisdom, or power, or danger. Others appear bathed in shadows, no matter how much light is in the surrounding environment. Some people have a very stable energy. Without saying a word, they put you at ease, make you feel relaxed and calm. Others have a very unstable field. Within minutes—sometimes even seconds—you feel the restlessness of their energetic body, their instability, their "static" electrical condition. "He was nervous," we might say to a colleague or friend later on. "How do you know? Did you see him shake?" the friend might ask us. "No, but I could sense it," we say. Just as a lie detector works by measuring the electrical fluctuations within the body, so you and I react to the changes in another person's electrical field.

We are taught from childhood to censor such perceptions as irrational. Nevertheless, when someone sends out a powerful thought or feeling, you receive that thought or emotion—and very often make it conscious. Someone's sexual energy, for example, can be very strong and palpable, even when that person has made no overt advances. Violence and danger are other powerful forms of energy that emanate from the field and affect us consciously. More subtle waves of energy also radiate from the field, though we tend to reduce them to generalities. "I get good vibrations from this person," we sometimes say. Or, "I got really bad vibes." Yet, there is so much more to be gleaned from a person's field.

When we allow ourselves to observe the brightness of one person or the darkness of another, we recognize that the relative amount of light emanating has nothing to do with his or her complexion, or skin color, or hair, or clothes. Think of the auras of Nelson Mandela or Martin Luther King, both black men, and note the kind of radiant energy that emanates from them. Think of Mikhail Gorbachev, the Dalai Lama, John Kennedy, Pope John Paul, Mother Teresa, or Margaret Thatcher—all very different in coloring, complexion, and physical stature, but all radiating a powerful light that seems to shine far beyond their physical bodies. The energy field gives us all our power, abilities, and health.

Sometimes, we can actually see wisps of this energy, especially if a person is sitting against a white wall in normal indoor light, as if little flames of light were dancing around the person's head. If you allow your eyes to go slightly out of focus when you look at someone, the energy body will become even more visible. This occurs, in part, because letting the eyes go out of focus shifts the emphasis of sight to the rods, or those cells within the optic nerve that perceive low-intensity light. The counterparts to the rods are the cones, another group of cells within the optic nerve that perceive bright light and color. The auric field is a low-intensity light and consequently is more visible to the rods. Watch the energy move in flamelike patterns around the head and shoulders. It appears very much like hot pavement emitting heat on a hot summer day.

Another way to see the aura is to note the fragments of light and color that move around a hand or arm as the person makes a gesture. Sometimes, when the light is right, you can see the field chase after the hand, like gossamer light, as the person raises the hand to his head or lowers it to the table or the arm of the chair. The aura seems to be left behind as the hand moves, as if the hand were leaving a trail of light in its wake.

Your energetic field makes an impression on people, too. Though it is impossible to know exactly how you affect others, we affect those with whom we interact. As I will show in chapter 10, the field sustains personality characteristics and patterns of behaviors that can be positive or negative. These are energetic patterns, streams of energy or blockages that maintain our choices and behaviors. We also tend to attract similar kinds of people into our lives over and over again. If you reflect on the similarities among the people you attract and the consistency of certain of your experiences, you begin to see that these attractions are not coincidences but are responses to nonverbal, energetic patterns, messages we transmit. Healing touch can strengthen patterns—if we regard them as positive—or change behaviors—if we want to be free of them.

The Soft Resilient Field: A Model for Understanding

Think of the field as having the consistency of a big ball of cotton candy. In health, the field is soft, pillowy, and resilient. Each filament of energy within the field is like radiant spun sugar. Unlike the cotton candy, however, the filaments in the field are uniform and in perfect relationship to each other.

Shaped like an egg, the energetic *you* is a sphere of energy that surrounds and fills every cell of your corporeal body. The energetic body also extends about two to four feet beyond your physical form. It is radiant with all the colors of the rainbow. It is this energy that people are referring to when they use the word *aura* or talk about an auric field. The energetic you maintains your physical health and, indeed, the life of your physical body for as long as you are on this earth. According to the healers and mystics of both East and West, the energy body does not die when the physical body dies. Just the opposite: When the energetic body decides that its purpose on earth is complete, it leaves the physical body to return to the energetic or spiritual world. At that moment, your physical body ceases to function and returns to the earth as disparate elements. The consciousness that you know to be the real you, the "I" inside of you, lives within the energy body, which lives on eternally.

Chakras: Wheels of Energy

Embedded within the field are seven wheels of energy, known traditionally as *chakras*. These chakras are arranged vertically in the center of your body, from the base of your pelvis to the top of your head. Each chakra provides life force to a specific set of organs, tissues, and eventually to an endocrine gland. In addition, each chakra is a center of consciousness, providing emotional, psychological, and spiritual capabilities to the body, mind, and spirit.

The chakras are energy tunnels that swirl uniformly, like eddies of water. These perfect tunnels of energy are widest at the outside of the field and then funnel into the body to an endocrine gland. At the point where the chakra intersects with the body, it is about the size of your palm. At the endocrine gland, the funnel reverses itself, becoming larger and wider as it swirls from inside the body, out the back, to the outer reaches of the field. The chakra tunnel does not disturb the uniformity and flow of the energy fibers or filaments in the field but actually feeds them and helps to maintain balance and order within the field.

The seven primary chakras are located in the following locations (see diagram 5): the first chakra is found at the base of the pelvis and is known as the root chakra; the second is located at the center of the lower abdomen, about three or four fingers below the navel, and is called the sacral chakra; the third chakra is located at the solar plexus; the fourth chakra is located in the center of the chest, and is known as the heart chakra; the fifth chakra is located at the throat and is known as the throat chakra; the sixth chakra is found between the eyes, just an inch above the eyebrows, and is known as the chakra of the brow, or *ajna;* the seventh chakra is found at the top of the head and is known as the crown chakra. (For more on chakras, see chapter 5.)

In addition to these seven primary chakras, there are secondary chakras located on the palms of the hands, the backs of the knees, and the soles of the feet, and twenty tertiary chakras on the tips of the fingers and toes.

Seven Layers of Life

The energetic body is composed of seven layers. Each layer corresponds to a specific aspect of consciousness. The layers have a certain density that becomes more diffuse as you move away from the physical body; it is more dense and palpable as you move closer to the physical body.

In health, there is good communication among the layers of the field, so that each level influences the other six. All seven levels of the energy field are intimately connected and interdependent on each other (see diagram 6). For example, thoughts create emotions (and emotions create thoughts). Indeed, one cannot have a thought without the production of hormones, which can trigger emotional changes. The quality of that thought will determine the character of the emotion and the physical response we experience. Memory can

DIAGRAM 5. THE SEVEN CHAKRAS

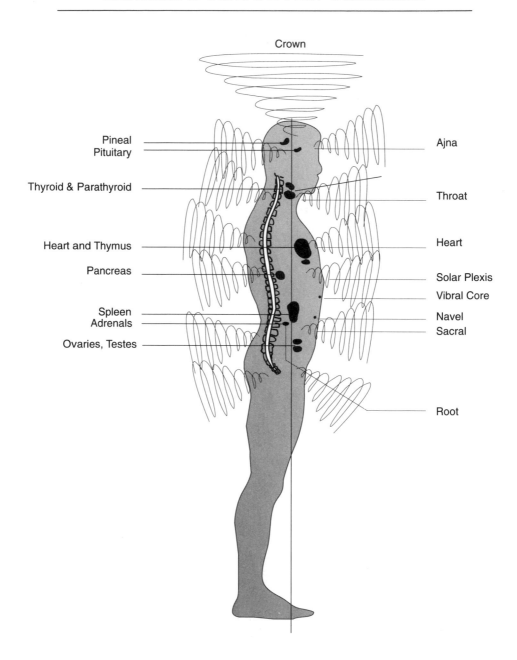

DIAGRAM 6. THE SEVEN LAYERS OF THE ENERGY FIELD

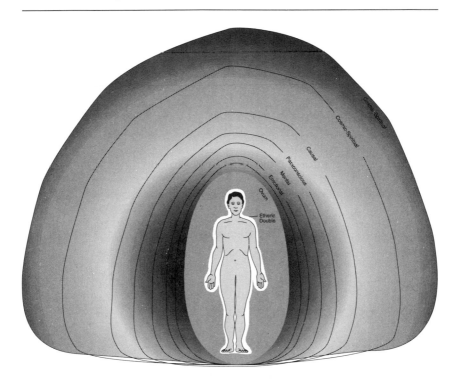

elicit compassion, fear, or emotional pain, all having different effects on the physical body as well as on various layers of the field. Because of this interaction within the field, you and I are able to experience a wide array of information at the same time. We can have an intuitive insight, for example, while, at the same time, we process that information intellectually and experience the joy that such a revelation brings. In this way, insight and joy give us a true sense of our direction.

The seven layers of the energetic body are as follows:

The First Layer: The Etheric Body

Often referred to as the aura or corona, this layer of energy is joined directly to the physical body. Every cell, tissue, and organ is infused with the ovum or etheric body, receiving the life force from this most intimate part of the field. The ovum or etheric body is often depicted in spiritual art. Another image that I often use to describe the etheric body is the waves of heat that come off a road on a hot summer's day. This ovum holds to the physical body and moves around it in much the same way, and is the easiest part of the field to perceive with your touch. All you have to do is hold your hand within a few inches of a person's body and you can perceive its powerful radiant energy. Whenever you kiss a baby, your lips perceive this layer in the field; often, a baby's etheric body is so palpable that it seems to have an almost liquid quality.

The etheric body, which extends between two and six inches from the body, is often referred to as the "etheric double" because all the organs are replicated in the etheric form. Indeed, your entire body is a physical manifestation of the etheric body. Rudolf Steiner, the German philosopher, writer, and psychic who created the Waldorf schools and Steiner medicine, said that all the physical organs are formed out of their exact replicas in the etheric body. The physical heart, for example, is formed out of the etheric heart. Your heart is an exact double, even a product of, the etheric heart in your auric field, which continues to send life force to the physical heart for the lifetime of the organ. All organs of the body are similarly nourished by the etheric body.

People who suffer an amputation frequently experience "phantom limb" phenomenon, which is the feeling that the hand, arm, or leg that's been lost is still present and can even be felt. The missing limb is indeed present in etheric body, and even provides vibrational feedback to the rest of the auric field, giving the faint physical impression that the missing limb exists. (It is this same auric field that is responsible for instructing salamanders to regrow amputated limbs, as cited in chapter 1.)

Humans are not the only living creatures with an etheric body. All plants and animals have the same corona, or golden glow, surrounding and permeating their every cell and fiber. The golden aura captured on Kirlian photography is this etheric body that surrounds the physical form. This is the part of the field that, in humans, salamanders, and all other living things, directs biological functions.

The Second Layer: The Emotional Body

From this level within the field, all our emotions, desires, joys, pains, sufferings, and passions emerge. Emotions are a form of radiant energy without physical form. The astral body and its emotional nature are common among all animals. Indeed, the lower or primitive aspects of our emotional or astral body link us with the animal kingdom. Yet, as Steiner and others have pointed out, only humans have an ego, the "I" that serves to organize all our human characteristics—including emotions—and subject them to higher levels of consciousness. We are required by this higher organizing center, the "I," to integrate our emotions, desires, and passions with the higher levels of our energetic field as well as with the physical body. As we all know, this is one of the most challenging aspects of life.

Emotions affect the body through the nervous, endocrine, muscular, and immune systems. Indeed, as every teenager quickly learns, you cannot experience an emotion without an instantaneous glandular reaction. Each emotion appears in the field as a charged constellation of energy. Depending on its nature and quality, an emotion can emerge within the field like a flower opening to the sun or like an explosion that showers the field with ecstatic or destabilizing energy. If the emotion is joy, the field opens and expands, sending energy radiating throughout the entire electrical and physical body. Immediately, the body experiences a flood of life force; every pore seems to open to the sun. The light within you is expanding, brightening, and opening up to the infinite energy that surrounds you and is channeled through your energetic field. In this moment, you are more alive than ever because you are experiencing love—the love of the universe for you!

That energy, that love, is always present, but changes in the field—caused by beliefs, perceptions, attitudes, and most of all, fear—cause the field to shut down or be injured. But when the moment of joy arrives, you open and experience the light that is all around you. The part of you that opens, specifically, is your heart, or your heart chakra, a whirling flower of energy over your heart. You experience this opening and are filled with the light of love, which in turn floods your field and your physical body.

The healing that can take place in that moment can be miraculous. Depending on how much life force is penetrating your field and physical body, that love can overcome barriers or forms of stagnation that are currently causing physical symptoms and disease. Love, hope, joy, and feelings of well-being—all of these are generators of energy within you that cause the field to expand and open, and result in similar openings within the physical body.

You have experienced the electrical quality of emotion hundreds—even thousands—of times. Think back to your first date, the first time you touched the hand of a boy or girl whom you liked. Something tangible, electric, and altogether wonderful passed between you. Think back to your first kiss. Need I say more?

If, on the other hand, the emotions are negative, the opposite effects take place. Small to moderate degrees of anger or conflict cause the energy within the field to become erratic. It is an irritating energy that causes similar nervous, muscular, and hormonal irritations in the body. Great anger, fear, or hatred wound the field, causing rifts, holes, walls between layers, and great storms of energy within the field that wound even further. When an angry patient arrives, the field feels to me as if it is hard and pushing outward, as if it is pushing people away. Anger also causes the field to have jagged edges, as if it contains knives that are being fired at me. Frenetic, unfocused energy, on the other hand, feels like static electricity, or little spikes of energy.

Changes within the field cause immediate changes within the body. For example, the well-known fight-or-flight reaction occurs when fear stimulates the adrenal glands to secrete adrenaline, which in turn becomes epinephrine, dopamine, and norepinephrine, chemicals that trigger an incredible array of thoughts and physical reactions, among which are increased heart rate, respiration, blood glucose, and muscular activity. Fear depresses immune response, increases heart rate and respiration, and causes heightened muscular activity. If the fear becomes chronic, cholesterol levels are elevated significantly, hormones—especially catecholamines—become heightened and imbalanced, respiration becomes shallow and tense, and muscles remain tense and sometimes go into spasm.

Conversely, positive emotions—such as love, hope, joy, and feelings of well-being and security—all strengthen immune response and make the physical body better able to fight off disease. In this case, the emotions are smooth and flowing. What most people do not realize is that these changes—both positive and negative—originate in the electromagnetic field that surrounds and permeates the body, and that many come from the astral layer of the field.

Emotions, of course, are directly linked to our thoughts, which exist in the next level up within the energetic field. Even unconscious emotions—those emotions whose sources still lie unrecognized in the unconscious—create thoughts of which we are conscious. For example, we may be angry at someone and have long internal monologues with ourselves, yet never realize the deeper reasons for our anger; perhaps we are really angry at ourselves or at someone whom the person in question reminds us of. Indeed, it isn't until the emotions and thinking work in harmony— that is, until our emotions are allowed to emerge and our thoughts are made free to investigate the sources of these emotions—that we understand our emotional world.

All of us have experienced the "energetic" nature of emotion, though we find it hard to use words to describe the experience. For example, remember the last time you were embarrassed. This emotion, which we usually try to keep hidden, nonetheless causes a variety of physical responses: the ears and face redden and become hot, the scalp may twinge a little, and our hands may begin to sweat. We experience palpable changes in respiration and heart rate and, overall, we shrink just a little. Shame, another powerful and negative emotion, often causes the face to become pale and the whole body to physically fold upon itself. Again, we feel ourselves shrinking energetically, as if we were being drained of energy. Guilt is another emotion that we experience as a kind of wound in the heart; at the same time, we experience an inexplicable loss of energy.

The loss of energy that occurs whenever we experience guilt, shame, or unresolved anger is referred to as a *leak* in the field. The boundary that maintains the integrity of the field is torn. Through that tear, energy leaks and is lost. We experience guilt as a loss of integrity, personal protection, and a blurring of our own boundaries. We are no longer capable of protecting ourselves from another person's judgment of us. It's as if we have absorbed another person's assessment and made it our own. The boundary that supports our sense of self is injured, allowing energy to be lost. We experience a palpable diminution of the life force, with all its familiar and well-known weaknesses: fatigue, self-condemnation, loss of direction, and a weakened sense of self. Anyone who has ever witnessed a child being yelled at by a parent or some other adult has seen the child react as if he or she were being hit. The child may visibly recoil in an attempt to escape the verbal and energetic blows.

For the healer, the emotional layer of the field is an essential part of the healing process because most illnesses are very often rooted here. Old traumas and long-standing emotional wounds will appear as areas of dull thick energy, like stones or boulders or scar tissue. Often, I experience blocked energy on the astral plane as having an almost tarlike viscosity. For more recent wounds, you may experience patches of heat or swirling, active, even pulsating energy. (I'll talk more about the specific feelings associated with blockages later in this chapter and farther on in the book.) When the practitioner of therapeutic touch begins to work with these stagnant forms of energy, all the old emotions will begin to emerge at first, though with less intensity. Recipients of healing touch may re-experience events that took place long ago or find themselves thinking of specific people or situations that were forgotten or repressed. Unexpected images can come to mind, even for the practitioner while he or she is performing healing touch. Eventually, if healing touch is continued, the person can be freed of these memories and emotional blocks. The energy can flow smoothly again and healing can occur.

After the healing touch session is complete, a meditation or guided imagery can help the person repattern the emotional plane. This will help close wounds and establish new and healthier habits.

The size of the astral field is determined by the emotions, thoughts, and intentions of the person in question. People deal with emotions in so many different ways, but among the most common is to repress them, which has a shrinking effect on the field. Also, people who are driven by selfish or egotistical motives tend to have smaller, darker energies on the emotional plane. You will feel such a person's energy field as thin, close to the body, and insufficient to hold another person's feelings, hopes, or desires.

Rudolf Steiner offers an insight into the power of love to affect another person's energetic field. He states that whenever you maintain a loving thought for someone, such as when you are conducting a session of healing touch, your thought escapes your own energy field as a "form of light" in the shape of a flower, which enters the person it is intended for in the astral and etheric fields. It then directly strengthens the recipient's field, causing increased vitality, health, and happiness. Simply sending a thought of love has this effect, says Steiner, no matter what the distance between you and the person you wish to help. Thus, energy work is accomplished no matter whether or not you use your hands. Often, your intention alone is sufficiently powerful to change another person's condition.

The efficacy of one person's healing thoughts on others, even those at a considerable distance, has been demonstrated in many scientific studies. Randolph Byrd, M.D., a cardiologist, used a computer to divide randomly a group of 393 coronary patients at San Francisco General Hospital into two groups. Group 1, which was composed of 192 patients, was prayed for each day by a separate group of people who came from a variety of religious faiths. The members of group 2, composed of 201 patients, were not prayed for. No one connected with the study—including the patients, doctors, and nurses—knew who was being prayed for and who wasn't (this is called a double-blind study). As for the people who prayed for group 1, each member of the prayer group received the first name of several patients, along with descriptions of the patients' condition. That meant that each member of group 1 had five to seven people praying for him or her each day for the ten-month study period.

The findings, published in the *Southern Medical Journal* (July 1988), were so startling that they convinced even many hard-core skeptics. After ten months of following both groups, Dr. Byrd and his colleagues found that the patients who were prayed for were five times less likely to need antibiotics (evidence of improved immune function) and three times less likely to develop pulmonary edema (a condition in which fluid fills the lungs as a consequence of inadequate pumping of the heart). None of the members of the prayed-for group required endotracheal intubation, while twelve of the members of group 2 required the procedure; and fewer members of group 1 (the prayed-for group) died.

Other studies that have examined the influence of prayer have shown similar results. Like healing touch, prayer has been shown to affect the health of plants, fungi, and bacteria. Research has demonstrated that people can use prayer effectively to inhibit the growth of fungi, even at a distance of fifteen miles.

The power of prayer demonstrates the importance of your intention while you perform healing touch. In short, send those you work with your love and make your healing touch sessions an act of prayer.

The Third Layer: The Mental Body

The third layer of the field is responsible for intellectual function, the conscious and unconscious mind, and many memories. The conscious mind, of course, refers to those aspects of ourselves and our environment of which we are aware. By unconscious, I mean the personal unconscious—those thoughts, memories, and dreams that have been repressed or forgotten but that exist just beneath the surface of our consciousness. Higher layers of the field relate to the archetypal world, elucidated by Plato, Swiss psychiatrist Carl Jung, and others.

The mental body coordinates physiological activity, including conscious and autonomic functions. It gives you the ability to, say, drive your car many miles while you think of everything but driving and yet arrive safely. Biofeedback and relaxation techniques allow a person to gain access to the mental body and to make unconscious and autonomic functions conscious and accessible to mental control. Dr. Krieger, a nurse researcher at New York University, and others have demonstrated that during a healing touch session, both the practitioner and the client experience an increase in the production of alpha brain waves, the electrical patterns associated with deep states of meditation. Such alpha states are associated with deep relaxation, slowed heart rate and respiration, and expanded perception, including experiences such as extrasensory perception.

Among the important contents of the mental body, especially from a healing perspective, are the unexamined ideas, beliefs, judgments, and concepts that give rise to our behavior and can inhibit our growth. Beliefs, judgments, and attitudes that no longer serve our current state of maturity and development exist as blockages to circulation of energy within the field. They stand rigidly in the way of new information, fresh insights, and larger belief systems. Like boulders in a stream, or knots of tension in muscles, they block circulation of energy within the field, preventing renewal and new understandings of life. Even worse, these unexamined judgments and beliefs feed the conscious mind and cause behaviors that are inappropriate to our current situation. They prevent us from seeing situations in a fresh, new light. Racism, sexism, and various beliefs of superiority or inferiority are all examples of blockages in the mental plane. Beliefs that you are weak, or talentless, or "always wrong" (or "always right") are also unexamined judgments that impede health and development. The insistence "I can't do that" is an unchallenged belief that becomes energetic patterns in the field. These patterns prevent the free circulation of energy within the field, which limits our freedom and our creativity and affects our health.

Many psychological projections reside here in the mental layer. An example is the person who projects the notion that powerful people are ultimately selfish and seek to prevent him or her from rising to higher levels of responsibility and success. People who insist on being victims of every difficult situation, or those who try to manipulate others because they fear being forthright or honest in their relationships, are commonly blocked on the mental plane.

As a practitioner of healing touch, you will release these blockages from your loved ones' or clients' fields. When that occurs, you will frequently hear people start talking about their frustrations, their projections, or their unexamined beliefs from a whole new perspective. Some will have revelations of how they have limited themselves. Others will simply feel tremendous relief or a new sense of personal power and identity.

Once some of the long-standing beliefs are released, far more creativity emerges. Great relief and flexibility are felt. The person feels empowered simply because he or she has been unshackled of beliefs that have prevented him or her from seeing the vast array of possibilities—and opportunities—implicit within situations.

The Fourth Layer: Paraconsciousness

Jack Schwarz, author of *Human Energy Systems* (E. P. Dutton, 1980), calls the fourth level the layer of paraconsciousness. The fourth level contains all the extraordinary abilities, such as intuition, extrasensory perception, image projection, spiritual sight, and clairvoyance. In addition to these abilities is one's capacity for compassion. Rudolf Steiner maintains that one form of intuition is the ability to join with another person, to feel his life condition, to know his pain and suffering. Out of such intuition comes compassion for another human being.

Here, Steiner gives us an insight into how intuition actually works. Intuition is the ability to experience the true connection that exists among all people—and indeed with the Great Spirit or Tao or God. When we experience that unity, we open ourselves to the information that is passing constantly through the cosmos in the form of energy. On a one-to-one level, you can experience connectedness simply by listening and feeling another person's life force. Various forms of Oriental diagnosis teach methods of developing intuition by allowing the client's energy to contact your own field so that you are able to touch your client's energy body with your own field. In this way, you can understand the person in a deep and intimate way. (In chapter 7, I provide methods and exercises for doing this, as well as ways to release any of your client's energies that you might have picked up during your session.)

We practice this awakening to connectedness whenever we perform healing touch. During a session, the practitioner channels universal energy through himself or herself to the client. The practice is based on the fundamental unity among the cosmos, the practitioner, and another human being. By doing this, you are living in the awareness of connectedness, which accelerates the development of your intuition and the fourth level of the field. No ESP or clairvoyance or spiritual sight is possible without a deep connection to the oneness—either with another person or with the cosmos itself.

Your ability to allow your intuition or the fourth layer within your field to guide you depends on how clear and unobstructed the lower layers currently are. By removing obstructions from these levels of our being, the fourth and higher layers can influence the mental, emotional, and etheric bodies. Consequently, our feelings of connectedness and intuition automatically improve.

The Fifth Layer: The Causal Body

Traditional approaches to the field maintain that there is a place within all of us that knows why we are here on this earth. This layer of the field contains the knowledge of your life's purpose, your many talents, and the lessons you wish to learn while you are on this earth. The causal layer contains the knowledge that awakens in you, if only faintly, when you encounter people with whom you have agreed to work out specific tasks, accomplish goals, and overcome barriers before you came to the earth. On this layer of the field, your soul's plan for this lifetime can be found.

Virtually all religions have taught that reincarnation, or the transmigration of souls, is the foundation of life. This is true of Buddhism, Taoism, early Christianity, and the Kabbalistic teachings within Judaism. We live multiple lifetimes on this planet so that we can learn and evolve to higher states of being. In the process, we accumulate knowledge, which we use in each succeeding lifetime to help ourselves and others. In addition, we make mistakes and incur karmic lessons, or debts, that we wish to propitiate. All of this is done so that we can develop greater and greater love, knowledge, and understanding of the meaning of life. Life itself is an inextinguishable resource; it cannot be destroyed, and so continues to manifest in the forms that best replicate the consciousness associated with that particular life form. The physical body perfectly replicates the consciousness of the being within it, and serves to manifest in physical form all the abilities and lessons that each individual soul wishes to experience, express, and learn. All such information about your individual lifetime, as well as all previous lifetimes, is contained within the causal body, the fifth layer of the field.

Traditional spiritual and religious beliefs have taught that expressing your innate abilities, working with those people with whom you have made spiritual and karmic agreements, and learning the lessons that you came into life to learn are the sources of your greatest joy. All of them combine to move the spirit closer to its ultimate goal: complete union and harmony with God, Tao, the

Great Spirit, or whatever name you wish to call the source of all life.

It is important to recognize that you do not have to believe in reincarnation to serve as a practitioner of healing touch. On the contrary, all you have to do is to care deeply about the person you are trying to help and to serve as an instrument for the universal love and energy that will pass through you to the person you wish to help. There need be no greater understanding or conceptualization than that.

The Sixth and Seventh Layers:
The Cosmic and Spiritual Consciousness

The sixth and seventh levels of our beings represent our most intimate links with what each of us recognizes as God, the Great Spirit, or the universal creative force. Obviously, all aspects of the field and the physical body are directly linked to the divine universe, but the sixth and seventh layers actually *know* it and are consciously in direct contact with it. Consequently, these layers offer us the experience of direct union with God. They sometimes are able to resonate within our consciousness when we are deep in prayer and meditation. It is this level of our beings that is being experienced when a person is said to have a momentary enlightenment.

Not much is known about these levels of the field, simply because they are so rarefied and lofty that very few people consciously experience them and then write about their experiences. What we do know is that the sixth and seventh layers of the field possess a tremendous force of energy that, when it grounds in the body, can create a host of psychological disorders if the person is not prepared for such an experience, or if the body itself is not in sufficient health.

The Dead Sea Scrolls lend credence to this theory and point to the fact that the early Hebrews were well aware of the power of these upper levels of the field. The scrolls were produced by a sect of Jews called the Essenes, who ventured out into the desert, to a place called Qumran, where they prepared for the coming of the Messiah. One of the ways they prepared was to observe strict dietary

laws that conformed to their traditions. But some scholars maintain that the Essenes also were purifying themselves with the intention of creating a familial line of great constitutional strength; such
a family would eventually produce a son whose physical powers
were sufficient to hold the energies of the sixth and seventh layers of
the field.

It is well known that the Essenes placed great emphasis on the
physical constitution of every member of their sect. They believed
that a person's physiognomy, or physical characteristics, could be
read to discover the spiritual development of that person. The Messiah was to possess the purest physiognomy, reflecting both his
great constitutional strength and his spiritual inheritance. Rudolf
Steiner also maintained the same belief, writing that the Hebrews'
strict dietary and lifestyle laws enabled them to produce a body that
was capable of carrying the sixth and seventh layers of the field, or
the Christ spirit.

Layers Interact with Each Other

In order to better understand the topography of the field, I've described the layers individually, but this separation does not reveal
how the layers interact, influence each other, and function as one.
While each layer of the field has its own unique function, strengths,
weaknesses, talents, and abilities, it must work in coordination with
the entire field in order for us to express our talents and abilities and
learn about life. The person who has a gift for music is using his or
her entire field while playing an instrument, clearly beginning with
the physical body and including the first layer (the etheric body, to
coordinate the voice or the muscles used to perform on an instrument), the second (placing the depth of feeling in the music), the
third (providing the intellectual ability needed to learn the music
and express it with nuance and precision); the fourth (experiencing
music's power to unify people in harmony and sound), and the fifth
(music is part of a particular person's life plan and expressing that

plan provides the greatest of joys). If the musician truly reaches great heights, he or she has the potential to express the divine sound—or, as Pythagoras called it, the "music of the spheres." All the layers of the field must work in harmony if the person is to truly express his or her gifts.

The Central Tube: The Channel of Spirit in You

After several years as a practitioner of healing touch, I realized that in addition to the standard layers, there is another characteristic of the field, which I call the central tube (see diagram 7). This tube, or channel of energy, runs down the center of the physical body itself. It originates at the very top of the head, where the spiritual life force enters the body, and runs down the center of the body through the neck, down the center of the digestive system, to the very base of the sex organs, where the energy can pass out of the body and where the earth's energy can enter into it. Along the tube are found the seven wheels of energy, or chakras, each of which fan out and enrich the organs in that particular area of the body. This is a kind of spiritual channel running from top to bottom.

Energy runs like a river through this tube. Blockages within the tube often appear as eddies of energy and can prevent energy from flowing cleanly through this essential channel. The most frequent problem I have found among those with blockages in the tube are emotional conflicts, specifically the problem of integrating concepts of the head with the emotions and instincts of the heart and lower organs. As we will see in chapter 5, specific aspects of consciousness are located within the seven chakras that are located along the tube. The chakras represent (among other things) specific aspects of our human psychology. People who have great difficulty integrating the head, the heart, and the sexual-survival instincts often have blockages in the tube. Life force that would otherwise flow smoothly among these three centers is blocked, causing the mind to behave as if it were separated from the emotional and

DIAGRAM 7. THE CENTRAL TUBE

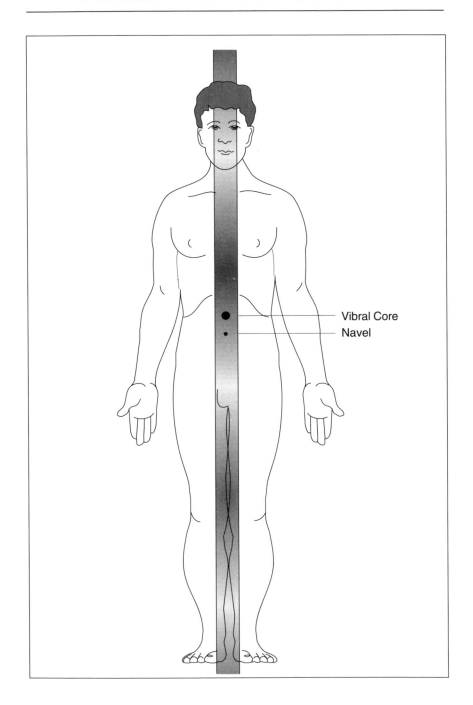

Vibral Core
Navel

sexual-survival centers. Such a person is continually in conflict over what he or she thinks versus what he or she feels or secretly wants, or is instinctually drawn to.

By eliminating these blockages, we can help the person integrate the higher and lower centers of the psyche and restore the brightness and clarity of the mind.

In the center of the body, just below the solar plexus and just above the umbilicus, is the center of being, known as the *vibral core*. Here, spirit and matter join and become one. This is where the vital healing energy flows from the practitioner to the client. The energy originates from the creator of the universe but flows to the practitioner, who sends it forth from the vibral core. Thus, healing energy flows from the universal source to the practitioner's vibral core, then to the practitioner's hands, and then to the client's vibral core. Twylah Nitsch maintained that the vibral core is where the father spirit (energy) and the mother earth (matter) mingle to create our essential humanness. When the healer and client work together, their energetic bodies mingle and become one. That oneness is established between their vibral cores. This vibrational union harmonizes the two people and directs both of them in the healing process.

The Body Is the Product *of the Field*

Most of us believe that health and illness reside entirely in the physical body. Indeed, all of Western medicine is based on this fundamental belief. Hence, the principal forms of treatment in the modern armamentarium are drugs, surgery, and radiation—all directed exclusively at the physical body. Ancient and traditional healers stand this belief on its head. Our ancestors taught that the physical body is the *creation* of the energetic field, which itself is part of the larger spiritual world. In the same way, health and most forms of illness begin in the energy field and ultimately manifest in the physical body. There are exceptions to this, such as when we are exposed to a toxic chemical or a pathogen in the environment. But even these examples are not so clear-cut as you may believe. Your ability to ward off a chemical or pathogen depends to a great extent on the strength of the energetic body, which supports your immune system and organs of elimination. When these systems and organs are functioning optimally—thanks in part to a powerful life force— you are able to avoid many of the toxic side effects of modern life. This, of course, is demonstrated every day, as some people effectively ward off the toxic effects of their environments while others do not.

In the vast majority of cases, the physical manifestation of disease is the last stop in a process that began in the energetic field. Whenever a blockage manifests in the field, life energy is prevented from flowing optimally to the body or to a specific place within the body. When numerous blockages manifest, the flow of life force is diminished. As I have said, without life force the body cannot survive. Without optimal life force, the body cannot sustain health.

There are many reasons why blockages or other types of injuries to the field can manifest. Psychological and/or physical trauma commonly injure the field. Many such energetic wounds can be healed, however, unless a belief system sets in that supports the continued existence of the wound. The most damaging belief, of course, is fear. All of us have beliefs that support our fears. We believe that certain types of people or situations are particularly threatening. Or we believe that we are inadequate to handle certain conditions in life. Such beliefs change our behavior and alter the energetic field that supports our lives. They cause us to develop patterns of energy within the field. These patterns eventually manifest as blockages, or tears, or even leaks—wounds that prevent us from experiencing our own boundaries and allow our life energy to drain from the field (I'll discuss patterns of energy, blockages, and leaks in greater detail in chapter 7). In any case, strong beliefs—and especially fear—are usually at the bottom of all illness. For example, a certain person works too hard because he believes that unless he works seven days a week he'll fail to please his superiors; perhaps he believes he'll be fired or he'll be broke. In the end, his fears and his excessive work manifest as imbalances in the field that prevent life energy from flowing to the body, which in turn contributes to illness. Someone else is afraid to experiment with life, fearing that any deviation from the "tried and true" will lead to mistakes or "sin" or retribution. Thus, she never comes to know her true nature, desires, and abilities. Ultimately, such a rigid approach to life contributes to frustration, anger, and disease.

Yet, sickness should never be seen as a punishment for mistakes or imbalances. All of us become sick and all of us will die and none of the illnesses that we encounter is regarded by traditional healers as "punishment" for anything you or I might have done. We may speculate as to why one person became ill, or why another died in this or that way, but such speculation is just that: It is a guess, a hunch based on partial information, which leads inevitably to inaccurate conclusions. As Paul wrote so eloquently in 1 Corinthians (13:12): "For now we see through a glass darkly; but then face to face: now I know in part, but then shall I know even as also I am known." Remembering that we know only in part is a good exercise in humility, especially for a healer. Practitioners of healing touch are not so interested in knowing why people become ill as much as we are in addressing the blockages in the energy field.

Ultimately, sickness is a mystery that each of us must confront and derive our own conclusions and enlightenment from. Sickness and health hold their own unique gifts that we must discover for ourselves. On the higher spiritual levels, illness is another way to develop greater understanding of life and compassion for ourselves and others.

The Real You Behind Your Eyes

Susan, a fifty-year-old married woman with two children, came to me in 1986, overweight and suffering from edema, yeast infection, allergies, swollen hands and feet, and a swollen, distended stomach. She had skin rashes, was regularly fatigued, and was often irritable and depressed. She also suffered from regular insomnia. Susan had followed numerous weight-loss programs with no lasting effect. She kept losing and regaining the same twenty-five pounds. As for the skin rashes, she applied topical ointments that provided temporary relief but no lasting cure.

When Susan first came to me, I placed her on a diet that would eliminate many of the foods to which she had intolerances or sensitivities. But her previous experience with diets had made her resistant to yet another regimen. I usually wait until after the diet and nutritional therapies have strengthened the underlying organs before I begin a program of healing touch, but in Susan's case I decided to start early in our treatment program.

"After the first couple of energetic treatments, I started to feel better," Susan said. "The first thing I noticed was that I slept better and I was generally more relaxed. What was surprising was that I also began to feel better about myself. I started to have a better sense of my own power. I didn't know why I had these benefits. All I knew was that I felt better. And I was certain my improvement had to do with the therapeutic touch."

Shortly after Susan began seeing me, her husband suffered a heart attack. This occurred right before Christmas, and the stress of that event hit her family like a tidal wave. "After my husband had the heart attack, he had a triple bypass operation. Naturally, we were all upset. I went to Deby a lot then to help me relax and get me through the crisis. It was amazing how helpful this practice was to me. I really felt something good happening whenever I had a session. I felt lighter, stronger, more relaxed. I was able to maintain a consistent positive attitude through some pretty rough times." It wasn't just her attitude that was improving. All her physical symptoms, including the edema, the yeast infection, and the rashes, were disappearing.

Because Susan felt she was benefiting so much from the practice, she had me perform healing touch on her whole family, including her husband, Don. "Deby did therapeutic touch on him right up to the time he went in for the operation," recalled Susan. "It made his outlook brighter, more positive. It built him up, made him stronger before he went in for the surgery. After the surgery, Deby did therapeutic touch on my husband's leg where the surgeons removed the vein that would be used for his bypass graphs. Normally, the leg would become swollen and painful, but after therapeutic touch, he healed quickly and had no swelling or pain."

After several weeks of healing touch, Susan had no trouble following a healthy diet, which relieved her food intolerances and caused her to lose weight. Her weight fell to 125 pounds, which on her five-foot, five-inch frame was ideal. All the bloating left her, as did her yeast infections and the extended bouts of irritability and depression. Today, Susan has turned her experience with therapeutic touch into a new vocation. She continues to study this powerful healing tool and is practicing therapeutic touch at a local chiropractor's office two days a week. "One of the main benefits I received from healing touch was a big change in self-esteem. The longer I do this practice, the stronger I feel. I just feel better about myself. I used to be a housewife and a mother, and when my kids got bigger, I started to feel that there was nothing left for me to do. This practice gave me a bigger view of myself and I realized that I could help people with it."

Like many people who begin practicing therapeutic touch, Susan soon discovered that she could actually experience the energy field that surrounds all of us. "When I'm working on someone's foot, let's say, I can feel the energy coming off the person's foot. Sometimes it feels like I'm lifting the energy off and away from the foot.

"It takes a certain leap of faith to begin using this practice, but as soon as you commit to doing it, your confidence grows because you can see and feel the very tangible results."

EXERCISES

Here's an exercise that you can perform during early evening—it's best at twilight—that will help you see the auric field around your hands. Turn off all artificial lighting and lie on your back on the floor. Raise your hands a foot or so above your head and join your fingers in a relaxed weave. Now, very gradually pull your hands apart so that your fingers gently and slowly separate as your hands move in opposite directions. As your hands slowly separate, relax your focus gaze between your hands so that you are looking at the space between your hands and at the ceiling of your room. Slightly blur your vision (as I explained in a previous section). You will likely see streams of soft light between your hands and fingers. The light will appear much like vapors that surround your hands and dance between your fingers.

As discussed earlier in the chapter, ask a friend or partner to sit in a well-lighted room against a pale or white wall. But instead of just concentrating on the field, carry on a conversation with the person. While you are looking at him or her, slightly blur your vision while you gaze at the light around his or her head and shoulders. Note the wispy quality of the light. It seems to move in flame-like motifs around the person's head. Also note whether the quality of the wisps change as you converse.

Often, we have trouble experiencing energy because we identify exclusively with the body. Here's a meditation that can help you see yourself as more than your body, more than your emotions, and more than your intellect.

MEDITATIVE ALIGNMENT EXERCISE
(Attunement)

1. Sit in a chair or on a pillow on the floor with your back straight and your body comfortable and relaxed. Breathe deeply and establish a deep rhythmic pattern of breathing (Breathe in a

regular pattern for approximately one to three minutes). Slowly draw your attention away from your environment and focus on the in and out movement of your breath. Let go of all your thoughts.

2. Bring your attention into your physical body. Take some time to notice where you are holding your tension. Breathe deeply and evenly into the tension and visualize the tension stretching out and becoming relaxed. See the area of tension becoming smooth and supple. Then say to yourself, I have a physical body and I am more than my physical body.

3. Now bring your attention into the emotional body. Take some time to become aware of your feelings. Take a personal inventory of what is going on within you. Notice your feelings; do not judge them or try to change them. Then breathe into those feelings and visualize yourself letting go of them; see them fade from your consciousness and say to yourself, I have an emotional body and I am more than my emotional body.

4. Move your attention into your mental body. Take an inventory of your thoughts. Notice the amount of activity going on in your mind. Breathe deeply and slowly and quiet the mind. Release all thoughts and arrive at a place of stillness. Take a moment to experience the stillness, then say to yourself, I have a mental body and I am more than my mental body.

5. Focus your attention at the top of your head and say to yourself, I am a center of pure creative awareness and higher spiritual will. Allow yourself to fully experience that statement. Feel its power and the grace that flows to you from this recognition.

6. See yourself as an energetic field, a living energy, that has consciousness and love. That love flows to you from an infinite source; it can never be extinguished. You can send that energy to others to help them in endless ways, including helping them to heal. Say to yourself, I am in the flow of power. I am a channel of power and that power is love.

EXERCISE
Feeling the Field

1. Stand face-to-face with your partner at a little more than an arm's distance from each other.

2. Extend your arm directly out from your side, toward your partner's shoulder, but still well back from your partner. Keep your elbow bent slightly.

3. Cup your hand loosely and gradually bring your hand toward your partner's shoulder.

4. As your hand approaches your partner's shoulder, move your hand slowly through his or her field, slightly raising and lowering your hand a few inches, so that you can delineate the various layers and densities of the field. Feel the field with your hand. Note the changes in thickness, temperature or patterns as your hand perceives as it moves through the field.

5

🕉

The Chakras:
Spheres of Energy,
Consciousness, and Life

If you take your hand and place it gently over your heart, allowing your fingertips to touch your shirt ever so lightly, and then slowly rotate your hand in a clockwise direction, as if the clock face was sitting on your chest with the numbers facing outward, you will feel comforted. If you continue to rotate your hand in that gentle, circular way, you will feel your body relax and get warmer. Gradually, you will likely experience a strange communion with this part of your body, as if your heart area were smiling at you in gratitude. Breathe deeply and allow that smile to warm your entire inner being. Many people who do this exercise eventually start to cry. They cry because they feel comforted, relieved, and overwhelmed with gratitude, as if they were being welcomed into a realm in which all their burdens could be put down, a realm in which they were embraced by an unconditional love. (Try doing this exercise by reversing the motion of your hand over your heart. Note the difference in the feeling.)

When you do this exercise, you are applying healing touch to your heart chakra, the sphere of energy that governs your heart and thymus gland and a specific realm of your consciousness. In doing this exercise, you get a small glimpse of the unity of your body, mind, and spirit. You also recognize that you have the power to gain access to your spirit and influence it in healing ways. As you progress through this book, you will learn many other techniques for healing your body, mind, and spirit through simple yet powerful methods of healing touch.

For the practitioner of healing touch, a knowledge of the chakras is an indispensable diagnostic tool. The chakras also are the sites at which great healing can occur. We can understand people according to their chakra imbalances, but more important, we can do so much for them by working with the chakras through healing touch. Finally, the chakras demonstrate the importance of your intention, for your intention reveals the chakra from which you are expressing yourself. As we have seen, your actions will have very different effects on the recipient, depending on the chakra by which you are motivated. If you, as a healer, are acting from your heart chakra, you are channeling the energy that can utilize all your other abilities—the furthest reaches of your mind and your deepest, most practical wisdom about survival. Ultimately, the chakras prove what the poets have always taught: that the greatest integrating and unifying force in life is love.

The information I provide here on the chakras comes from my own experiences and from numerous other investigators in this field, especially from Swiss psychologist Carl Jung, spiritual teacher Ram Dass, and numerous experts on Sanskrit, Ayurvedic healing, and traditional Eastern Indian spirituality.

Chakras: Where the Body, Mind, and Spirit Are One

Nothing illustrates the unity of body, mind, and spirit better than the chakras. *Chakra* is a Sanskrit word meaning "wheels" or "circles of movement." The chakras are spirals of concentrated life force—vortices of energy, as they are referred to by some. They are arrayed in a straight line on the front of your body, starting at the very base of your spine (at the perineum) and extending to the top of your head. The seven primary chakras are located as follows: The first is found at the base of the spine; the second a few inches below the navel; the third at the solar plexus; the fourth over the heart; the fifth over the throat, at the larynx; the sixth between the eyebrows; the seventh just above the crown of the head. Each of the seven primary chakras radiates downward into your physical body and outward through the seven layers of your energy field. Each chakra is shaped like a cone or a spiral, with the pointy end entering the body and the ever-widening end spiraling outward into your energy field.

In addition to these primary chakras, you also possess smaller, secondary chakras on the palms of your hands, the backs of your knees, and the soles of your feet near the arches. There are even smaller tertiary chakras located on your fingertips and on the toe tips. You use the second and third chakras in your hands to direct energy during healing touch, and you use the second and third chakras in your feet to ground yourself while performing the practice.

As you will notice shortly, the function of each of the seven primary chakras corresponds roughly to the seven layers of the field, so that the activities of the first layer of the field (the etheric layer) correspond to the first chakra; the second layer of the field corresponds to the second chakra; the third layer with the third chakra, and so on.

One of the functions of the chakras is to act as funnels for the life force. Each of us is continually bathed in an unlimited flow of electromagnetic energy, or the life force that sustains our lives. We breathe in the life force, receive it through the five senses, channel it through the field, and draw it into us through the seven chakras.

The chakras can be understood on several levels. On the gross physical level, they channel life force to particular organs and endocrine glands. Indeed, when you look at the illustration of the chakras (see diagram 8), you'll notice that they correspond with the most active parts of the body—the brain, eyes, speech center, heart,

DIAGRAM 8. THE CHAKRA LOCATIONS

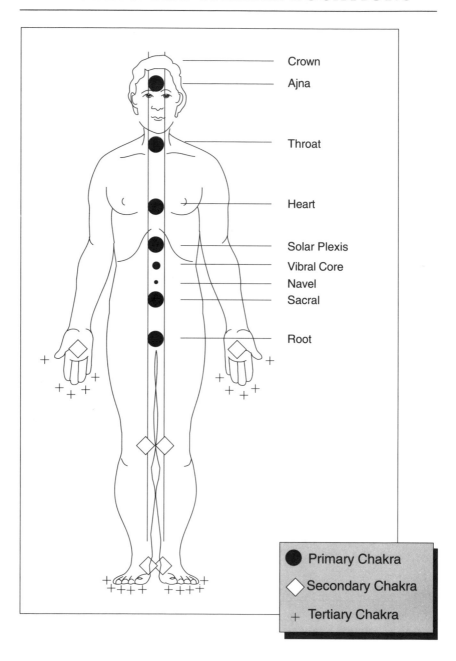

Crown

Ajna

Throat

Heart

Solar Plexis

Vibral Core

Navel

Sacral

Root

● Primary Chakra

◇ Secondary Chakra

+ Tertiary Chakra

middle organs, digestion, endocrine glands, and sex organs. These areas, obviously, require a great deal of energy. But we can say the reverse as well: that in their enormous activity, these same areas of the body generate the most energy. These are the parts of the body that give rise to thoughts and ideas that, in turn, shape our world; they recall memories that sustain relationships; they drink up light and color; they masticate and digest food; they pump and cleanse the blood; they procreate and sustain life. In short, they are the basis upon which we experience life—and even participate in its creation. Little wonder, therefore, that ancient sages correlated these parts of the body with special vortices of energy that would sustain such important functions.

But there is much more to these chakras than the purely physical. These seven zones also carry with them profound emotional and psychological associations, of which virtually all of us already are aware. For example, on some visceral and well-established level of our knowing, each of us regards the heart as the center of the emotions. We say about some people "He has a lot of heart" or "She has the heart of a lion" or "He's a heartless soul." To express our deepest love, we might say "I give you my heart." Other chakra areas possess their own unique character and associations: the brain, for example, is regarded as the realm of intelligence, objective thought, and reason, even though the brain is directly linked to virtually every physical, psychological, and emotional aspect of our humanity. When trying to assess a person's character, we search his eyes for insight into his soul. We look at a person's bloated and enlarged stomach and on some intuitive level wonder if he's not perhaps a slave to his appetites. Sigmund Freud became a giant by articulating just some of the associations we have about sex and our sex organs. (Even Freud did not elucidate all that we know and believe about sex.) And as we all know, our associations with each of these areas go beyond the physical, energetic, and psychological. They bring us into the realm of spirit.

In fact, each chakra is the site of a specific consciousness, a realm that offers its own specific set of values. None of us has integrated all seven levels of consciousness into our being. You may be awake and motivated by two, three, or even more chakras, but it is the very rare being who is awake and functioning at all seven levels of consciousness.

Which brings me to an essential point. The one, two, or three chakras that might be most influential in your life dictate your physical and emotional needs, your values, and your spiritual awareness. The world today is being governed by the first three chakras. As a species, we are now struggling collectively to break into the fourth chakra and allow its values and consciousness to direct our lives and permeate our world.

The chakras, therefore, represent a kind of ladder of personal, psychological, and spiritual evolution. Each of us is attempting to move into the next higher chakra above the ones that now direct our worldview. Hence, the values and awareness implicit in the chakra that we are striving for represent our next step in growth and development. The chakras describe in ascending order how we proceed from the very rudimentary consciousness to an ever-enlarging viewpoint on life and ourselves.

As we will see, moving up the chakra ladder inevitably presents the greatest challenges life has to offer. Very often, one or more of the chakras are blocked or partially closed. That means that we are not being influenced sufficiently by the corresponding values and understanding that reside within that chakra. It will also mean that the life force will be diminished in that part of the body. Yet, even when one or another chakra is closed, it still functions in some limited capacity. It is still providing nourishing life force to its corresponding part of the body. If the chakra did not function on some level, we would soon be dead. Still, when a chakra is operating in a weakened state, the part of the body to which it corresponds is also weakened. In addition, the values and consciousness represented by that chakra do not influence us as strongly, if at all. Gradually, the related organs and glands may atrophy and eventually manifest some kind of symptom or disease. Also, our lack of understanding for the part of life represented by that chakra inevitably brings us into conflict and crisis.

By understanding a person's problems, and at which of the seven chakras he might be fixed, the practitioner of healing touch can understand why certain physical and psychological problems manifest. The practitioner will also know which of the seven chakras the client is struggling to integrate into consciousness, and therefore where the practitioner must concentrate his or her work.

As a practitioner of healing touch, you are doing more than working on physical health. You are working with the body, mind, and spirit, and in so doing, you are treating the underlying reasons we become sick in the first place.

Let's turn now to an examination of the seven chakras individually and collectively to better understand their role in our lives and in the practice of healing touch.

The First Chakra: The Root of Being

Referred to in Sanskrit as the *Muladhara*, or the root chakra, the first wheel of energy is located at the very base of the spine and encompasses the perineum. It provides life force to the adrenal glands, which in turn produce adrenaline for instinctual and instantaneous responses to exciting events or perceived threats. This chakra provides life force to the large intestine, rectum, bones, legs, and feet. It is also responsible for maintaining the nervous and circulatory systems. Physical symptoms that emerge when this chakra is congested, blocked, or closed include constipation, hemorrhoids, obesity, sciatica pain, arthritis, knee trouble, anorexia nervosa, and suicide.

The first chakra is responsible for grounding your life in physical existence. It is your instinctual center, your energetic and spiritual root on the earth, the source of your survival instinct. It keeps you rooted in the present moment and aware of possible threats to your existence. Any reaction related to your survival, including the flight-or-fight instinct, emanates from this center of consciousness. Conversely, any self-induced threat to existence, such as anorexia or an attempted suicide, is a breach of the values and consciousness inherent in this chakra.

Kundalini yoga and Ayurvedic medicine teach that the first chakra is responsible for maintaining our sense of smell. The human olfactory sense is quite developed, though we usually don't think of ourselves as good smellers. In fact, we can identify an object after smelling just nine molecules of the particular substance, which means that we can often perceive something at a considerable distance from our nose.

Our faculty of smell was developed as a means of self-protection. Smell allows us to perceive whether or not something is poisonous or somehow dangerous without having to eat it, for example, or to get too close to the object in question. (Cautious children and adults invariably place unknown or foreign foods under their noses before they dare taste something that they might find revolting or dangerous.) This relates directly to the chakra's overall responsibility for survival.

There is an enormous body of literature and mythology surrounding the seven chakras, and much attention has been paid to the first chakra. Out of this mythology has come our understanding of the consciousness and values that lie within this wheel of energy.

To begin with, this chakra is associated with the earth and the color red. It is characterized by cohesiveness, inertia, and a certain amount of stagnation. The first chakra makes us cautious, which is a kind of inertia. It encourages us to remain focused on our number-one priority, which is survival. And it prevents us from allowing too many contradictory thoughts and bits of information to enter our consciousness, which would break down the mind into fragments. This is part of its character of cohesiveness.

The earth chakra is symbolized by a giant black elephant that is holding up the world. In his writings about the first chakra, Carl Jung stated that the elephant, placed as it is at the very root of existence, symbolizes the enormous power and strength that supports human consciousness. The elephant symbolizes how strong is our foundation. Without such a foundation, we would not have the confidence and spiritual strength to develop awareness of ourselves and of the world around us. Yet, because the foundation is so strong, said Jung, humanity has the security and even the yearning to expand its awareness and thus to grow.

Yet, the first chakra mitigates our curiosity and growth by making us constantly aware of our need to survive. The first chakra is Darwinian in its nature. Survival of the fittest is its law, which means its impulse is to see situations and people in competitive terms. Hence, this chakra's energy is one of separateness and individuality. People who are dominated by the first chakra live in constant fear for their lives. They may affect a secure manner, but they evaluate all information and all people on the basis of whether or not they are a threat to life, livelihood, and possessions.

Hence, the first chakra is the realm of your separateness from other living beings and, indeed, your separateness in the universe itself. From this chakra, we experience our aloneness.

The Second Chakra: Sex, Passion, and the Water World

Referred to in Sanskrit as *Svadhisthana,* or the center, the second chakra is located a few inches below the navel at the region of the first lumbar vertebra. It provides life force to the ovaries in a woman, to the testes in a man, and to their related hormones. The chakra channels life force to the male and female genitals, kidneys, bladder, and circulatory system. It also serves a developing fetus with life energy.

This chakra is also responsible for governing the sense of taste and the deep vital breath. According to Chinese medicine, the kidneys make the deep breath possible. When the kidneys are strong and vital, they draw the breath deep into the bottom of the lungs.

When the kidneys are weak, the breath is shallow and the person is timid, nervous, and fearful.

Blockages, closure, or any impairment of the second chakra can result in illnesses related to the kidneys, bladder, sex organs, and the lower back. All emotional and psychological issues related to sex emanate from the second chakra, including how one expresses oneself as a male or female.

The chakra's main biological functions are the maintenance of the sex organs, the sex drive, the desire for physical pleasure, and all the social issues associated with entering into a sexual relationship. One cannot truly experience sex alone, and consequently the second chakra leads us from the individualized state articulated by the first chakra into the search for a mate and the realm of social interaction.

The second chakra is regarded as the center of the personality. In Japan, it is known as *hara,* or the center of gravity. Hara is the foundation upon which one maintains physical, emotional, psychological, and spiritual equilibrium. It is the center of power and vitality, say the Japanese. From hara, one maintains balance—no matter what the circumstances—and therefore controls himself and his environment without lifting a finger. All the martial arts—whether they emerged from Japan, China, or Korea—are based on strengthening and sustaining one's center of gravity, or the second chakra.

The second chakra is associated with the color orange and the water element. It is symbolized by the leviathan, or sea serpent. What the elephant is to the earth, so the leviathan is to the oceans. It is the embodiment of the enormous power and mystery that lies beneath the intimidating surface of the seas. Water, of course, connotes fertility, the womb, and the bodily fluids that carry sperm and egg. It symbolizes the unconscious mind and its infinite mysteries that lie beneath its waves. Consistent with this image is the fact that water and the serpent represent a primitive stage in the evolution of life on the planet, when living creatures inhabited the oceans exclusively. In writing about this chakra in his book *Alchemical Stud-*

ies (Princeton University Press, 1967), Carl Jung wrote: "We are reminded of the 'days of Creation,' of the time when consciousness arose, when the primordial unity of being was barely disturbed by the twilight of reflection, and man swam like a fish in the ocean of the unconscious."

The ocean is the mother of life on the planet, the womb from which we all emerged. Indeed, while each of us was in our mother's womb, we underwent a reptilian stage that replicated our earlier journey from the ocean waters to land.

Mythologically, the serpent symbolizes consciousness and choices. It was the serpent who introduced Eve to the "tree of the knowledge of good and evil" and encouraged her to eat its fruit. Once she and Adam had eaten the proverbial apple, their eyes were opened and they became conscious of their surroundings and their nakedness. In other words, they were suddenly more aware of themselves and their environment than they had been before. They understood good and evil, though they might well have been too immature at the time to do much with that knowledge. Nevertheless, mythology has consistently revealed the serpent as the symbol of wisdom and consciousness. In considering the second chakra, Jung wrote that the serpent "is the power that forces you into consciousness and that sustains you in the conscious world."

The serpent, of course, is a sexual image, and it symbolizes the central function of the second chakra: sex, sexual gratification, and reproduction. But as we all know, sex is never so uncomplicated as to be restricted exclusively to a simple act. Sex, as Jung says, leads us inevitably into greater awareness of ourselves and of others because it leads us into the complex and often contradictory world of relationships between the sexes. Such contradictions, of course, force us to stretch our understanding and increase our awareness of ourselves and others.

According to Native American and ancient Greek mythology, the serpent also symbolizes transformation, healing, and rebirth. The Native Americans saw the snake's talent for shedding its skin as a transformative process by which a living thing is reborn. Greek mythology depicts Hermes as carrying the caduceus, which is the winged sword wrapped by two intertwining snakes. The image of the caduceus, long regarded as the symbol of wisdom and healing, was later adopted by the medical profession.

The second chakra is a step upward along the evolutionary ladder because it reveals that the human has taken care of his survival and can now consider sexual relationships and even procreation. Such relationships don't happen until after we feel sufficiently secure in our environment to go out and make friends. Or, as Ram Dass writes in *The Only Dance There Is* (Anchor Books, 1974): "See, you've got your security under control and now you start to go into sensual pleasure and sexual desires and reproduction. You can't be busy reproducing if you're protecting your life, but the minute your life's protected a little bit, then you can concern yourself with the next matter, which is reproducing the species." Ram Dass points out that Sigmund Freud is the master spokesman for the second chakra.

Thus, the second chakra is concerned primarily with sex and the behaviors related to having sex or entering into a relationship in which you can have sex.

The Relationship Between the First and Second Chakras

Let's pause a minute and reflect on the first two chakras and how their value systems affect our lives in very different ways. Since it is concerned with the preservation of life and of separateness, the first chakra makes us aware of the dangers of life and our own aloneness. That aloneness makes us aware of our incompleteness and our need for companionship, love, and sex, which means it drives us to the second chakra. In its truest form, the pursuit of the opposite sex is based on love.

Sexual love is the union of opposites, man and woman, yang and yin, heaven and earth. In all traditional spiritual and religious practices—but especially those of the East—human sexual experience is regarded as the union of divine opposites. It is seen as the way for humans to glimpse the harmony and order that occurs when two halves of the cosmic puzzle come together in love. In the ancient Hebrew and early Christian traditions, the fact that sex was so pleasurable was considered proof that God is good. In yoga and Tantric traditions, sex permits two people to reenact, and thus participate in, the coming together of archetypes, cosmic deities. It is one way humans can participate in the divine drama, which is essential in the creation of life.

On the most basic and fundamental level, however, sex overcomes separateness. If it is expressed with love, it overcomes loneliness, isolation, and independence as well. In sexual love, we recognize the interdependent nature of life. Thus, if we are to enjoy sexual love, the consciousness of the second chakra must overcome the consciousness of separation, which is to say, it must overcome the consciousness of the first.

The Third Chakra: Power, Mastery, and the Ego

The Sanskrit word for the third chakra is *Manipura,* or "gem center." It is located at the solar plexus, or the region of the eighth thoracic vertebra. The third chakra is responsible for providing life force to the pancreas. It also funnels electromagnetic energy to the liver, gall bladder, spleen, and stomach.

The pancreas, of course, is responsible for creating insulin, which makes blood sugar available to cells as fuel. The third chakra is therefore associated with metabolism and the basic work of the cells of the body. Metabolism is, in fact, a tiny fire inside the cells. Like tiny factories, the cells burn glucose (or blood sugar) so that they can do their work. Hence, the third chakra has traditionally been associated with fire—or, in Ayurvedic medicine, with the fire element.

Blockages or closure of the third chakra result in digestive disorders, ulcers, diabetes, hypoglycemia, liver problems, and disorders related to the metabolism of blood sugar and fat.

Psychologically and spiritually, the third chakra is all about your personal power and self-mastery. Personal power and mastery are developed because you are required to refine yourself and mature. Hence, you are required to embrace the third chakra. Ram Dass states that the supreme spokesman for the third chakra is Alfred Adler, the Austrian psychologist whose philosophy centered around power as the central theme in relationships.

In addition to fire, the third chakra is also associated with the mind and the color yellow. This chakra is represented by the ram, which is the symbol for the zodiac sign of Aries, known for its strong will, courage, outgoing nature, leadership, and, indeed, its stubbornness. Aries is often joined with Mars, the planet of fiery passions, war, impetuousness, emotion, assertiveness, violence, courage, and activity. This chakra provides you with the capacity to assert yourself and your wishes and the power to fulfill what you set out to accomplish.

Hence, the atmosphere of the third chakra is all about passion, raw power, and an untamed mind.

Yet, the chakra is symbolized by the ram. Carl Jung points out that the ram is a sacrificial animal. This symbol reveals how personal mastery and power are actually achieved: by sacrificing the wild passions that are inherent in this stage of consciousness so that discipline, order, and concentration can prevail. The raw and naked power of the third chakra can make one behave like a wild goat: unruly, undisciplined, egotistical, and selfish. Life demands, in fact, that these characteristics be brought under control. Inevitably, we are thwarted in our wishes and are required to refine our self-expression and skills if we are to advance along our path.

When we are deeply frustrated, we often feel physical pressure or unease in the solar plexus. The third chakra is alerting us to the fact that our passions are unruly and that our personal power is being blocked or frustrated, perhaps by our own beliefs, perhaps by circumstances in the environment, or perhaps by both. There are two courses that can be chosen at this point. Either we can self-reflect, be creative, and apply a new approach to the situation, or we can push harder and force our will. This can lead to more frustration, anger, and resentment, which is why the third chakra is often associated with violence.

The Relationship Among the First, Second, and Third Chakras

Clearly, a progression of consciousness can be seen from the first, second, and third chakras. Having confronted our separation and aloneness, we are driven to sexual relationships, which joins us with at least one other human being and thus leads us beyond ourselves and our own priorities. The third chakra leads us back to ourselves, this time focusing on self-improvement and self-empowerment.

In a sense, the third chakra is an evolved first chakra: Both the first and third chakras are interested in you, the individual. The first chakra is more concerned with your survival, while the third is more concerned with the power needed to fulfill your desires. Yet, there has been an evolutionary step in between the first and third chakras, a step represented by the second chakra.

The second chakra leads a man and a woman into a sexual relationship, which typically results in children. As every parent knows, children force an adult back on himself or herself. They require the parents to love and develop their talents and skills in order to provide for their children's needs and survival. Parents are stretched by the demands of family to raise their children with love, order, and understanding. They must discipline themselves and even postpone their own desires to provide for those in their care. Indeed, they must sacrifice their own needs, and sometimes even their own lives. Women lose their lives in childbirth. Yet, they welcome pregnancy. Fathers sacrifice the attention and maternal love of their wives so that their children can enjoy such love and attention and thereby develop fully. Fathers, too, give their lives for their children. Ultimately, love demands sacrifice and self-development, which means that the second chakra leads inevitably into the third.

In a fundamental way, awakening to the second and third chakras—indeed, surrendering to them—means opening up to the worlds above the third chakra, because sex and self-development involve us in complicated relationships that ultimately require love.

Confronting the Crisis of the Third Chakra

The third chakra encourages us to utilize our own power, to be responsible for our own fate. Thus, it pushes us to realize our talents, our individuality, and to achieve self-mastery. Such a consciousness leads us inevitably to one of two crises.

The first is the crisis of demagoguery. The paradox of self-mastery—indeed, one of its pitfalls—is that as people progress in their development, an inevitable ego inflation sets in. As they become more skilled, more successful, they also can become more arrogant. They can indulge in the false belief that they are masters of their own fate. This can ultimately isolate them and destroy their lives. That is only one of the dark roads that the third chakra can lead us down, however.

The second is the one most of us find ourselves on—the road that leads to grief, sadness, and self-recrimination for not having achieved all that we wished for. Here, at the third chakra, are found many of our frustrations with ourselves. By the time we reach mid-life, we often find ourselves asking very hard and critical questions, such as: Why didn't I do this, or become that? Why didn't I make better choices along the way? These questions precipitate a life crisis, very often a mid-life crisis, in which the imperatives of the third chakra—the overwhelming desire to become master of our own fate—force us to conclude that we have failed in life. We didn't master ourselves so thoroughly, we decide. We didn't become the great person we set out to be. Thus, very often we feel bitterness and grief, which becomes locked in the third chakra.

The healing of the third chakra depends upon our moving upward to the fourth, which beckons us to evolve to a higher point of view, to see life in larger terms. That growth step is a particularly difficult one, however, because our modern culture urges all of us to be independent, self-sufficient, and masters of our own fate. Our culture leads us to live according to the first, second, and third chakras. Yet, our healing lies in moving upward to the fourth.

It is love that leads us to the fourth chakra.

The Fourth Chakra: Awakening to Unity

Known traditionally by its Sanskrit name, *Anahata,* meaning "un-struck," the fourth chakra provides life force to the heart. The name of the heart chakra, Anahata, means to emit a cosmic sound that is heard beyond the realm of the five senses. It is a sound that is "un-struck," meaning it has no origin, yet it exists. Its location is the first thoracic vertebra, or the area of the heart. It also provides Qi to the thymus gland, the lungs, the arms, and hands. Problems related to the heart chakra manifest as symptoms in these organs and extremities, including heart disease, high blood pressure, asthma, and other lung diseases.

The central ethic of the heart is love in all its manifestations, but most of all as compassion. Compassion means caring for others, which leads to healing. Thus, the heart chakra is focused on altruism and improving the lives of one's fellow human beings. Healing begins with the heart, and healers themselves work from this chakra first if they are truly dedicated to helping others.

The heart chakra is the central conduit through which all the chakras express themselves. In this sense, the heart chakra is unique, but it demonstrates the universal need for love. Thus, all forms of healing, all forms of expression, all ideas, all information must be expressed with love and compassion if they are to do another person any long-term good. The heart chakra is therefore considered the matrix through which all the other chakras must express themselves.

Whenever a person's consciousness progresses from the third chakra to the fourth, he or she very often confronts some crisis in life. The reason is that the heart chakra, as I will explain shortly, brings about the most dramatic change in consciousness.

The sound of the heart chakra, Anahata, the "unstruck" sound of the cosmos, is the same sound that the Greek philosopher and mathematician Pythagoras called "the music of the spheres." It is a heavenly music that inspires and lifts the heart.

Tantric teachings refer to the fourth chakra as Purusha, "the essence of man," or the supreme man. In understanding the ideas and feelings associated with the heart chakra, one sees the ideal human being, or the Purusha.

In Ayurvedic medicine, the heart chakra is associated with the air element and the principle of touch. It is symbolized by the black antelope or gazelle, an animal known for its speed, lightness of being, and gentleness. Healing touch is done from the heart chakra.

From the heart chakra comes our ability to see the unity among people—indeed, the life we all have in common. As Ram Dass points out, the fourth chakra reveals to us that this shared life is, in fact, one life. From the perception of that shared life comes the recognition that what happens to you also happens to me. This brings compassion and the desire to work for the good of all people.

Everything that is understood in its unity and in collective terms comes from the heart chakra. Thus, Jung, whose psychology articulated the collective unconscious and the archetypal world, is a leading spokesman for the fourth chakra.

At this level of consciousness, the experience of our separateness and aloneness begins to dissolve. This is one reason why the fourth chakra is associated with air—because of its universality to human existence; indeed, its universality to all creatures that live on the earth. We all wish to avoid suffering and experience happiness. We all want to breathe the good air and receive what we need. Without this recognition, we are reduced to an existence governed by the first chakra, which is to say, by the law of survival of the fittest. In this case, we are little more than animals.

The heart chakra unites people in the mystery of love. I say it is a mystery because love has an indefinable power to unify one person with another; to unify a family, a community; to embrace humanity as a whole. As love grows, its circle widens, so that the unity of life is experienced ever more deeply.

The Relationship Between the Third and Fourth Chakras

Crossing over from the third to the fourth chakra is an enormous step in evolution, and it's not an easy one, writes Jung. It is fraught with obstacles and sacrifices. The identity that we associate as our true selves actually serves as an impediment to this step in evolution. Crossing from the third to the fourth chakra is like going from a very personal and self-centered view of life to a universal view. This universal view strips away something that each of us defines as our uniqueness. In a profound way, each of us is attached to our separateness, our individuality, and our desire for personal power. The illusion that we can control life and ultimately master all that life brings to us is exceedingly intoxicating. That illusion reinforces our individuality—we don't need anyone else, we tell ourselves. We can do it on our own. This cowboy mentality is especially deep in American culture and, as we all know, is at the root of many of our most profound social, economic, and ecological problems. All of these issues spring from the first, second, and third chakras. I do not mean to suggest that we ever stop being responsible for our actions and our own happiness, but at the lower three chakras, we see our happiness as having to be attained through struggle with other people or against situations. We do not see the larger forces of life that support us in our path and, in fact, support everyone's efforts at fulfillment. I am referring, of course, to the presence of the divine in all our lives.

Within the psyche is a larger divine presence known by many names, the most utilitarian being the higher self. This higher self is your true guide in life. Jung points out that the higher self, or what he refers to as the psyche, is evolving at its own pace and according to its own organic plan, and consequently will force us to confront the next stage in development with or without the acquiescence of the conscious mind and its organizing center, known as the ego. In fact, the higher self often causes a shift in consciousness at the very moment when we least expect it. This invariably precipitates a crisis. We are forced to acknowledge the limitations of our current values and our worldview, which means that we must grow to a higher perspective, not because we necessarily want to, but because we must in order to reestablish equilibrium, health, and happiness.

Once the psyche, or the higher self, forces us to awaken to the need to grow and embrace a new set of values, we must also recognize that we are no longer in total control of our lives. Obviously, if we were in control, we wouldn't be facing the crisis that caused us to review our current values. Indeed, the crisis forces us to recognize that we are in some way inadequate to whatever it is that we are facing.

This would be crushing—and often is—were it not for the fact that such a crisis is usually joined with an awakening to a new set of values, often whispered to us as if from some other quarter of our lives. We pick up a book that makes sense to us. We listen to a lecture that inspires us. We talk to a friend or a teacher who points the way. In some altogether mysterious way, life opens a door and we walk through it. Or, to put it another way, life awakens us to the fact that the values of the third chakra are no longer sufficient to guide our lives, and now we must turn to the consciousness of the fourth chakra. In doing so, we turn to the Great Spirit for help, and in some subtle and often modest way, that help guides us out of the crisis. In the process, we become conscious of the fact that the resolution of the problem did not come out of our own power, or personal mastery, but came instead from some mysterious outside source of help.

For many people, this crisis, which is so common at mid-life, becomes the source of rebirth, because the movement from the third chakra to the fourth is often based upon the letting go of the illusion of our own omnipotence and the awakening of larger spiritual forces that shape our destiny and can be turned to for help. The rebirth invariably occurs because it is based upon a new faith.

As Jung says, this crisis that stimulates one's growth from the third to the fourth chakra brings with it the recognition that the "psyche is self-moving, that it is something genuine which is not yourself." That, says Jung, "is exceedingly difficult to see and admit. For it means that the consciousness which you call yourself is at an end." Or, as Ajit Mookerjee put it in his book *Kundalini: The Arousal of the Inner Energy* (Destiny Books, 1982), "You are no longer master of your own house." You must now recognize that something larger is within you and that the identity you recognize as yourself is subordinate to this larger entity. This recognition is transformative, because it is an awakening to the presence of the Great Spirit in your life.

Paula's Story: Imbalances of the First, Second, Third, and Fourth Chakras

The difficulties in making this step are apparent throughout our society, especially in those who suffer from chronic depression. A few years ago, I began seeing a thirty-eight-year-old woman, whom I will call Paula, who suffered from chronic fatigue, depression, and heart palpitations. She came to me because she did not want to take the antidepressant suggested by her therapist and because she was having trouble implementing the changes her therapist was recommending. She was stuck, and the depression seemed to be getting worse.

Paula presented a host of physical characteristics that revealed where her problems were located: her face was dull, expressionless; her shoulders were rounded; her chest was concave. In short, her heart chakra, which sends energy from the heart up through the neck and shoulders and lights the face, was exceedingly weak. Some experience—or set of experiences—had injured her heart chakra. Paula had a weak sense of her own identity and integrity, and therefore could not establish healthy boundaries—a first chakra issue. Her boundary issues also manifested in her overly active sex life. Paula had trouble discerning when and with whom she should have sex and whom she should avoid sexually. Paula had trouble saying no to people; she could be talked into things too easily, and consequently she was taken advantage of. The effect of her profligate sex life was to create an injury in her second chakra, over her sex organs, which felt to me as if it were tender and raw.

She also lacked will—a third chakra issue. When she became angry, it was usually after the fact, and she wasn't able to express that anger to the appropriate person or in the appropriate situation. Instead, she turned the anger back on herself, injuring herself in the process. That injury was especially acute in the fourth chakra, which I soon felt was lacerated and wounded.

I worked on Paula's entire field for a two-year period, seeing Paula two to four times per month. I did several things during each treatment. I began by moving through Paula's field, removing blockages throughout the field. I also concentrated on opening the secondary chakras in Paula's feet, which would allow Paula to feel more grounded, safe, and empowered. It would also improve Paula's ability to receive the supportive, uplifting energy that flows from the earth.

Then I attempted to remove blockages that were concentrated in her first and third chakras. These obstructions existed in the chakras like bundles of stagnant energy—or what I refer to as stones, or boulders. The boulders prevented the life force from flowing freely through these chakras, thus weakening the chakras and the consciousness that was housed there. The effect was to give her a very blurred sense of self, and because the first chakra was weak, her very survival was called into question, a common occurrence in people who are depressed.

I tried to remove the blockages in the first and third chakras by gently reaching into the area of the chakra with my right hand. As I moved into the chakra, I rotated my hand slowly in a counter-clockwise direction, as taught to me by my teacher, Twylah Nitsch. Twylah explained that this counterclockwise motion allows healing energy to penetrate the field. She further explained that once inside the chakra, I should reverse the motion of my hand, turning it clockwise, which would allow me to scoop out the blockages and pull them free from the chakra. Why must I turn my hand in these directions? I asked. All she would say is that this is how her grandfather taught her. My own experience has taught me that the counterclockwise motion provides the healer with a certain amount of power that enables the healer's hand to enter directly into the chakra and dislodge the energetic mass. At that point, the healer reverses the motion, that is, turning the hand clockwise, to move the energy in its natural direction and thus assist the chakra in eliminating the stagnant energy. When my hand was outside the chakra, I then visualized the blockage moving off my hand and into light to be transmuted.

Once this was done, I concentrated on sending healing energy to Paula's second and fourth chakras, the areas of her sex organs and heart, respectively. I finished each session by closing the holes and wounds that were in the field.

The effect on Paula was gradual but significant. In the early going, Paula told me that she had begun implementing the behavioral changes her therapist had recommended. This was something she had been unable to do before she started receiving energy work, and it reflected her growing sense of identity and self-empowerment. After a few months of therapeutic touch, her depression began to lighten significantly. "I felt that I could see the sunshine for short periods of time," Paula said. She started to have hope again.

These improvements increased steadily over a two-year period, until Paula was finally able to feel in control of her life and experience the lifting of her depression.

The Fifth Chakra: The World of Sound and Hearing

The fifth chakra, referred to as *Visuddha*, or "pure," is located over the throat, at the third cervical vertebra. It provides life force to the thyroid and parathyroid glands, as well as to the larynx, neck, shoulders, arms, hands, and ears. It is associated with the speech center and with hearing. Problems related to the fifth chakra include disorders of the thyroid and parathyroid glands, stiff neck, hearing impairment, colds, sore throat, tonsillitis, and all voice-related disorders.

The fifth chakra is the realm of communication. All forms of expression are under the influence of the fifth chakra. So, too, is the sharing and the synthesizing of ideas.

The fifth chakra is the transition into the world of ideas, symbols, and communication. The first three chakras are concerned with material existence and individuality. The fourth chakra represents a transition point into the higher realms, a doorway into the world of spirit. From the fifth through the seventh chakras, the levels of consciousness become increasingly focused on the matters of spirit and immaterial existence. Consequently, the consciousness of the upper three chakras is more and more rarefied, more subtle, and spiritual in nature.

Like the first and third chakras, the fifth represents a turning inward from the more altruistic and outgoing heart center. At the fifth chakra, the person moves into the inner world of energy, sound, and light—light, because words and ideas illuminate the darkness that is ignorance and show us the way to resolution of conflicts and reconciliation with one another.

The fifth chakra is associated with the element ether, which, according to Ayurvedic medicine, is the vessel in which all elements mix. The color associated with the fifth chakra is blue, and its principal concerns are sound, hearing, and communication. The animal that symbolizes this chakra is the moon-white elephant, a sacred mythological creature that represents the powerful and mystical base upon which the mind and the world of ideas are founded.

The quality of our communication—the temperament and meaning of our words—is a direct representation of our underlying consciousness. For most of us, the fifth chakra is the instrument of the first three chakras. If we are bound to the lower three chakras, we communicate from our separateness and our aloneness; we communicate from our needs for sex and for companionship; and we communicate from our will to power.

The consciousness of the lower three chakras is essentially dualistic, in that they make a clear distinction between you and me. They also tend to define people and situations as either good or bad. There isn't much gray in situations, nor is there much overlap in the recognition of people's needs. Consequently, there isn't much understanding. But once we enter the fourth chakra, our communication through the fifth becomes increasingly universal. Our words take on greater magnitude because they unite people in understanding and in love. People are no longer seen as necessarily good or bad, but as humans struggling to avoid suffering and find happiness.

The fifth chakra, however, has its own consciousness and values, which is the plane of energy and light. Words and sound are invisible. Their nature is immaterial, yet they move the material world and they change it. Words and sound are an expression of the spirit, and because words and sound have so much power, they give us a glimpse of just how powerful spirit truly is.

The word *Visuddha*, or "pure," indicates that the ideas and values native to the fifth chakra are pure and perfect and that those who reach the fifth chakra are able to express the purity and perfection of spiritual ideals. In his book *The Inner Life* (The Theosophical Publishing House, 1978), theosophist Charles Leadbeater wrote that those who reach the fifth chakra and embrace its consciousness are able to hear the heavenly sounds. Also, the communication of such people is guided by heavenly spirits. Such a person can communicate love, compassion, and a rare insight into spiritual truths.

The Relationship Between the Fourth and Fifth Chakras

The fifth chakra represents a new level of detachment unknown to the fourth. The heart chakra is still very much attached to the material plane, in that it cares so deeply for other people and for the life we all share. At the fifth chakra, one understands the impermanence of material life and can see clearly where permanence and infinite truths really lie. The fifth chakra represents the kind of detachment spoken of in Buddhism, in which the world is recognized as *Maya,* or "illusion." Hence, the crossing over from the fourth to the fifth chakra requires a further letting go of this impermanent world for the eternal world of spirit.

The Sixth Chakra: The World of Wisdom and Forms

Known by its Sanskrit name, *Ajna,* meaning "command," the sixth chakra is located over the forehead, slightly above the eyebrows, between the eyes. The sixth chakra provides life force to the eyes, much of the central nervous system, and the brain. It also funnels Qi to the pituitary and pineal glands, both endocrine organs located in the middle of the brain. These two glands work in harmony to support the individual and unified functions of the sixth and seventh chakras.

Most authorities say that the sixth chakra is associated with the pituitary gland, which is the master gland of the endocrine system. It controls virtually all endocrine functions and thereby influences the entire body, both in its everyday operations and in the body's growth and development.

The sixth chakra is said to control various states of concentration and consciousness. This is the realm of omniscience. Whenever someone breaks through to this level of consciousness, extrasensory perception, clairvoyance, visions, psychokinesis, and other paranormal experiences occur.

The sixth chakra is associated with the color indigo, according to Christopher Hills, author of the book *Supersensonics* (Destiny Books, 1975). Hills has studied and written exclusively on the chakras. The chakra is symbolized by Om, the cosmic sound. Om represents the alpha and the omega, the beginning and the end of all things. There are no elements associated with the sixth chakra, since it is beyond material existence. It is the world of cosmic law, harmony, perfect order, and vibration.

To better understand the sixth chakra, we should consider that the seventh chakra is the realm of undifferentiated oneness. In order for that oneness to give rise to creation, it had to bifurcate, or divide into opposites, so that it could create polarity, energy, and thus provide the underlying substance of the spiritual and material worlds. The sixth chakra is that realm of bifurcation and creation, where all things were created in their original perfection. At the sixth chakra, all paradoxes, all seeming contradictions, are harmonized. Yin and yang, man and woman, day and night, positive and negative—all opposites are brought together as one.

The sixth level is regarded as the archetypal world, or Plato's "world of forms." All seminal ideas exist here. It is said that the Godhead referred to in all religions is here at the sixth level, the realm of pure ideas. To tap into the sixth chakra means to glimpse the all-knowing and thus to have insight into the past, present, and future. For this reason, it is associated with intuition, ESP, and other parapsychological states of consciousness.

Thus, the sixth chakra is the world of perfect knowing, the world of wisdom. "The wisdom center (Ajna) shines with the light of Cosmic Consciousness and reveals the universe in its unified wholeness of being," says Mookerjee in *Kundalini: The Arousal of the Inner Energy.*

The Seventh Chakra: Oneness

The seventh or crown chakra is referred to in Sanskrit as *Sahasrara,* meaning "thousand," or the lotus of a thousand petals. It is located at the back of the head, slightly above the crown. Some maintain that it actually hovers above the head at this spot.

This chakra also nourishes the cerebral cortex and much of the central nervous system. Its primary function is to unify understanding and integrate all ideas and states of consciousness. The crown chakra is responsible for synchronizing all the human senses and faculties and thus making the world coherent.

Malfunctions that occur in the crown chakra manifest as depression, alienation, and the inability to learn or comprehend ideas, situations, and people.

The crown chakra is the transcendental state beyond consciousness, what the Buddhists call the Void and the Hindus call Brahmin. It is the ultimate oneness, the state beyond description.

The seventh chakra is associated with the pineal gland, an endocrine organ that serves to maintain mood, among other things. For centuries, mystics and philosophers regarded the pineal gland as purely a spiritual organ. They associated the gland with light, intuition, and truth. Indeed, many believed that the pineal gland was the so-called third eye, or the eye of intuition. Seventeenth-century philosopher René Descartes maintained that it was the seat of the soul. Yet, the organ remained a mystery to scientists, who until very recently thought the pineal had no function at all. New research has corrected that archaic assumption, however. The pineal gland, it turns out, plays an essential role in the maintenance of our circadian rhythms (biorhythms), brain chemistry, and mood. Remarkably, the pineal is, in fact, highly sensitive to light. When deprived of light, such as in winter, the pineal gland secretes abundant quantities of a hormone called melatonin, which consumes the chemical neurotransmitter serotonin. The brain uses serotonin to help create feelings of well-being, positive thoughts, and to enhance its ability to concentrate. It also is the chemical basis for deep and restful sleep.

When the pineal gland is deprived of adequate sunlight, it produces more melatonin, which in turn depresses serotonin levels. This results in a widely suffered disorder called Seasonal Affective

Disorder, or SAD. SAD is exactly that: a disorder in which people feel depressed, fatigued, and withdrawn. Most people who experience SAD suffer it in winter or when they are deprived of natural lighting for extensive periods. The cure is simply to increase one's exposure to sunlight or full-spectrum lighting. This causes the pineal to produce less melatonin, which makes serotonin levels rise and results in increased feelings of well-being, positive emotions, better sleep, and the removal of depression.

As for the pineal's reputation as the human third eye, even that remains something of a puzzle. According to *Atlas of Human Anatomy,* by Samuel Smith and Edwin B. Steen, "Some evidence suggests that it [the pineal gland] is a vestigial organ, the remnant of a third eye." Perhaps it was an organ that existed early in human evolution and there's more to the pineal function than we currently know.

The color associated with the crown chakra, says Hills, is violet, although many Eastern Indian traditions maintain that there is no color associated with the crown chakra. This chakra represents the ocean of life to which we all return. It is the ultimate and indefinable state of love and bliss.

The Energy Spiral
Harmonizing High and Low, Heaven and Earth

My experience has taught me that the system of Chinese acupuncture is absolutely correct in its assessment that life energy, or Qi, flows in channels, or what the Chinese refer to as meridians. But it does more than that. Energy also flows in spirals, or eddies, especially in the primary and secondary chakras. In addition, life force weaves among the seven chakras, connecting and unifying them into a fully integrated whole (see diagram 9).

As I mentioned earlier, each chakra provides a concentrated flow of life force to a specific part of the body. It also represents a particular type of consciousness that must be integrated into our being. Were it not for the spiral of energy, there would be seven

DIAGRAM 9. THE ENERGY SPIRAL

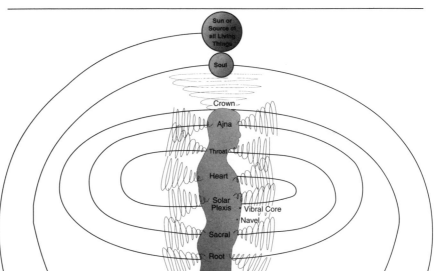

major subdivisions of consciousness operating in opposition to each other, much like seven heads of state running the same country. The net effect, especially on the physical and mental levels, would be chaos. Thus, the spiral of energy unifies the physical, psychological, and spiritual functions of the seven chakras and thus creates integration.

The spiral of energy has a distinct pattern, like a single line of threat that holds seven buttons in place on a shirt. The line itself begins at the heart chakra, emanating out of the heart and turning down and in to the solar plexus, or third chakra. There, it reenters the body and exits the back, where it loops upward and reenters at the back of the throat, or throat chakra. From the fifth chakra, or throat, the energy moves out the front of the body and loops downward into the second chakra, located in the area of the large intestines and sex organs. From there, it exits the back, turns in a semicircle upward, and reenters the body at the back of the head, at the sixth chakra, or third eye. From the third eye, the energy leaves through the front of the body and turns downward, again in a large semicircle, so that it enters the body at the root chakra, or at the base of the pelvis. From the pelvis, the energy arcs upward to the crown chakra, located at the top of the head. Within the crown chakra lies all the knowledge and life plan of the soul. Thus, the movement of energy through the chakra system is 4, 3, 5, 2, 6, 1, and 7.

Traditional people believed that the soul's journey on earth is already mapped out and that knowledge of one's life plan lies within each of us. Our challenge is to know ourselves and thus truly to understand why we are here on earth. The spiral of energy reveals this ancient wisdom in a very simple diagram. It shows that from the lofty heights of the crown chakra—the place where all self-knowledge lies—the energy turns downward to the earth, where the soul sojourns temporarily. From the earth, the energy spiral turns upward toward heaven, thus signaling our eventual return to our source.

Using the Energy Spiral as a Therapeutic Tool

This threadlike pattern unifies all seven chakras. It also joins individual chakras with their complementary opposites on the upper and lower parts of the body. Using the heart chakra as a center, we note that there are three chakras below the heart and three above. The spiral of energy begins at the heart and then weaves its way through each chakra, joining them in complementary pairs. For example, the root chakra, the lowest of the seven chakras on the body, is connected to the crown chakra, or highest, by the spiral of energy, thus joining the instincts to survive with the highest levels of ethics and universal love. The energy spiral exits the fifth chakra, located at the throat, and flows downward to the second chakra, thus unifying the voice and upper respiratory tract with the intestines, kidneys, and sex organs. From the second chakra, the energy turns upward to the sixth, or third eye, linking the lower intestinal function with the head and brain.

The energy spiral can be used as a diagnostic and therapeutic tool. If a client suffers from chronic headaches, I do not concentrate exclusively on the head and the area of the sixth chakra, but turn to the second chakra as a possible source of trouble. Very often, headaches have their source in the lower intestinal, kidney, and sex organ functions.

If a person suffers from chronic sore throats, a fifth chakra problem, I consider two other possible sources of the problem, neither of which are located in the throat. The first may be the area of the third chakra and middle organs—small intestine, lungs, liver, spleen, and pancreas. The third chakra provides life force to the fifth chakra via the energy spiral. If the third chakra is blocked, the fifth chakra will be deficient of Qi and will begin to manifest disharmonies. Dryness of throat, laryngitis, weak or breaking voice, accumulation of waste and mucus, and sore throat are common when Qi is deficient in the throat. In general, there is a feeling of emptiness in the field here; the person himself may experience this as weakness in the throat or lack of personal power. Therefore, when working on someone with chronic sore throats, I always clear the third chakra area, especially if there are chronic physical problems here as well.

On the other hand, the fifth chakra sends life force via the energy spiral to the second chakra, the area of the intestines, kidneys, and sex organs. If the second chakra is blocked, energy will build up in the throat, causing irritation, a buildup of mucus, the swelling of glands, and excessive heat.

The second possible cause of sore throats is repressed anger, held by the heart chakra (the fourth chakra). It must be remem-

bered that physical illness often needs to be treated pharmacologi-
cally, which may include the use of an antibiotic or herbs. However,
in order to truly heal a chronic sore throat—or any other disharmony in the body, for that matter—the underlying energetic imbalance must be treated. In the case of a sore throat, this means using
healing touch to treat the second and fourth chakras. In addition, I
also work on the chakras directly above and below the affected
area, which in this case would include the sixth chakra.

A recent client of mine, whom I will call Sally, is a good example of how the spiral of energy can be used as both a means of
diagnosis and guidance for treatment.

Headaches: When the Cause Isn't Just in the Head

Sally, forty-five-year-old wife and mother of two, suffered from
regular headaches, migraines, overweight, and severe premenstrual
syndrome (PMS) that included nausea and night sweats. Her gynecologist believed that Sally was entering perimenopause, which he
felt brought on the night sweats and nausea. The physician further
believed that the estrogen and progesterone Sally was taking to
alleviate the perimenopausal symptoms was actually exacerbating
her headaches. Sally was stuck. She didn't know whether to give up
the hormones, which would allow her perimenopausal symptoms
to flare, or to maintain the hormones that control the symptoms but
fueled the migraines.

Unfortunately, her headaches and migraines were getting
worse. She had to do something and eventually she came to me.

I saw Sally weekly for one year, during which time we made
remarkable progress. The first thing that healing touch gave Sally
was greater confidence in herself and a deeper sense of stability. She
started to talk about her own behaviors that might be contributing
to her problems, and by our third session together she realized that
her headaches came on after she ate certain foods, which she immediately gave up.

By the second month of treatment, Sally's headaches were less frequent. By the third, her migraines were gone. Over the next five months, Sally experienced only one migraine.

One of the first things I noticed as I worked on Sally's field was that the energy around her second chakra, located over the lower abdomen and responsible for providing life force to the sex organs, kidneys, bladder, large intestine, and adrenal glands, felt irregular, as if the chakra did not have an integrated consistency. I felt clearly that this part of her field was swollen, while other areas were weak or even withdrawn, as if there were a gaping hole in the field. As I continued to work on her, I kept getting the image of an open wound over the area of the second chakra. This corresponded with the physical problems Sally was having in her sex organs and adrenal glands. Even more telling was the fact that this part of Sally's field seemed even more irregular and swollen to me whenever she had headaches.

From an energetic viewpoint, this made perfect sense, since the second and sixth chakras are related through the spiral of energy. Clearly, the source of her headaches was the imbalance in the area of her second chakra.

Whenever I saw Sally, I worked on her second and sixth chakras first. I sent energy to the second chakra and then closed the wound by moving my hands in a very gentle pattern, as if I were literally bringing together tissue that had been torn apart. Then I turned my attention to the sixth chakra, which was congested and blocked. Here, I drew energy away from the chakra, opened it up, and increased the circulation within this part of the field.

After a few months of treatment, the wound in the abdomen seemed to be less swollen and starting to heal. At the same time, Sally's headaches and perimenopausal symptoms clearly had been relieved.

It wasn't until the tenth month of treatment that Sally began to lose weight—now without effort. This happy circumstance coincided with what Sally experienced as a dramatic shift in consciousness. She reported feeling better able to express her needs. She had always had great difficulty asking for emotional or psychological support. She was a big giver, thinking that if she was loving and supportive of others, that same love and support would come back to her. Often, it didn't. Also, Sally had a hard time setting boundaries for others. Thus, she ended up feeling taken advantage of and being trampled on. As a form of compensation, and a way to relieve her tension, she overate. Now she felt much stronger in herself. Sally found herself asking for help or saying that she simply could not perform certain tasks at home or at work because she was already too busy. At times, she said she marveled at her newfound strength.

By the time we stopped our regular work together, Sally was steadily losing weight. She was far better able to handle the stress in her life and her headaches were infrequent to rare. Though Sally decided to continue to take estrogen and progesterone, she suffered only mild symptoms of perimenopause. Her migraines had disappeared.

The Chakras

CHAKRA 1—ROOT CHAKRA

LOCATION	Base of spine, perineum
GLANDS	Adrenals
ORGANS	Legs, feet, bones, large intestine
FUNCTIONS	Survival, grounding, life promoting, vital physical energy
MALFUNCTIONS	Constipation, hemorrhoids, obesity, sciatica, arthritis, knee trouble, anorexia nervosa

CHAKRA 2—SPLENIC OR SACRAL

LOCATION	Two to three fingers below navel, lower abdomen, first lumbar vertebra
GLANDS	Ovaries, testicles

ORGANS	Uterus, genitals, kidneys, bladder, circulatory system
FUNCTIONS	Assimilation, life promoting, emotions, sexuality, desire, and pleasure
MALFUNCTIONS	Kidney/bladder trouble, female and male organic and emotional sexual problems, lower back problems

CHAKRA 3—SOLAR PLEXUS

LOCATION	Eighth thoracic vertebra just below notch where ribs come together to form xyphoid process to navel
GLANDS	Pancreas, adrenals
ORGANS	Liver, spleen, stomach muscles
FUNCTIONS	Willpower, personal power, taking in of energy from outside of self, growth, healing
MALFUNCTIONS	Digestive troubles, ulcers, diabetes, hypoglycemia, liver disorders, fat metabolism

CHAKRA 4—HEART

LOCATION	First thoracic vertebra, heart
GLAND	Thymus
ORGANS	Heart, lungs, arms, hands
FUNCTIONS	Self-love, love toward others, taking in life nourishment in general, mental energy, consciousness, healing
MALFUNCTIONS	Heart disease (including high blood pressure), asthma and all lung disease

CHAKRA 5—THROAT

LOCATION	Third cervical vertebra
GLANDS	Thyroid, parathyroid
ORGANS	Neck, shoulders, arms, hands, ears (hearing)
FUNCTIONS	Communication, expressive energy, volition, will (discernment and power of choosing), synthesizing of symbols into ideals

MALFUNCTIONS   Thyroid problems, hearing problems, stiff neck, colds, sore throats

CHAKRA 6—BROW OR AJNA

LOCATION   First cervical vertebra in back (space between and slightly above eyes on forehead)
GLAND   Pituitary (working in harmony with pineal)
ORGANS   Eyes
FUNCTIONS   Seeing, intuition, synthesizing
MALFUNCTIONS   Headaches, vision problems, nightmares

CHAKRA 7—CROWN

LOCATION   Top of head and slightly back where soft spot on baby's head is located
GLAND   Pineal (working in harmony with pituitary)
ORGANS   Cerebral cortex, central nervous system
FUNCTIONS   Integration and understanding
MALFUNCTIONS   Depression, alienation, inability to learn or comprehend

A knowledge of the anatomy and physiology of the chakras and their relationship to the physical body is essential in the practice of healing touch. The chakras offer the healer a set of portals into the body, mind, and spirit of the person on whom we are working. These portals are concentrations of energy and, indeed, of life. Within the chakras are the roots of many old wounds, blockages, and patterns that must be released if healing is to occur. Thus, the chakras offer the healer not only insights into the person's past but great opportunities to assist the person's rebirth.

EXERCISE—THE CHAKRA SPIRAL
(refer to diagram 9)

1. Envision a beam of rainbow light coming out of your heart in an arc and entering your solar plexus.

2. See the light pass through the solar plexus out the back, curve upward, and enter the body at the back of the throat.
3. See it pass through the throat and arc downward into the second, or sacral, chakra.
4. Envision the light passing through the body at the second chakra, exit the back, and turn upward and reenter the body at the back of the head, at the third eye, or sixth chakra.
5. Through the front of the third eye, see the beam of light arc downward and enter the body at the first, or root, chakra.
6. Visualize the light passing through the root chakra, exiting the back, arching upward, and reentering the body at the crown chakra.
7. From the crown chakra, see the light moving down through the center of the body to the bottom of the feet.
8. Once the arc touches the bottom of the feet, envision your entire field being lit up by the rainbow light so that the field is radiant with color and light.
9. From the feet, send an arc of light to the earth.
10. From the earth, see the light re-enter your body in the feet and turn upward, exiting the crown chakra and returning to the source of light and life.
11. Feel the rainbow light fill up every cell, tissue, and organ of your body with radiant light. Each organ absorbs the colors of energy that it needs for health and vitality.
12. When you feel full of light and life, open your eyes and let your light shine. If you become fatigued or imbalanced at any time of the day, you need only breathe in this radiant light to be restored.

If you tape these meditations with your own voice and play the tape to guide you through these mediations, your healing will be more profound.

Part Two

The Hands-On Practice

Disease [is] not an entity, but a fluctuating condition of the patient's body, a battle between the substance of disease and the natural self-healing tendency of the body.

—HIPPOCRATES

BUILDING THE ENERGY BALL

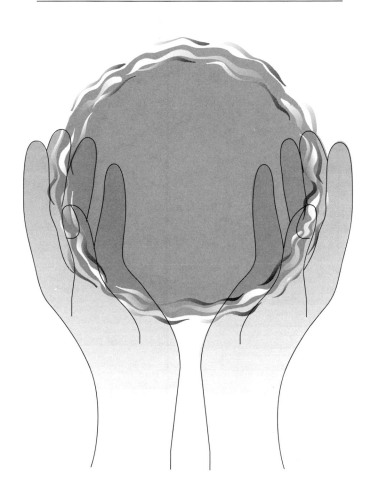

TRANSFERRING OF ENERGY
TO SHOULDER FROM ENERGY BALL

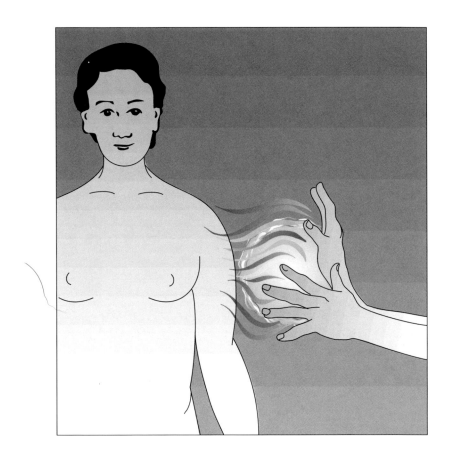

ENERGY FIELD

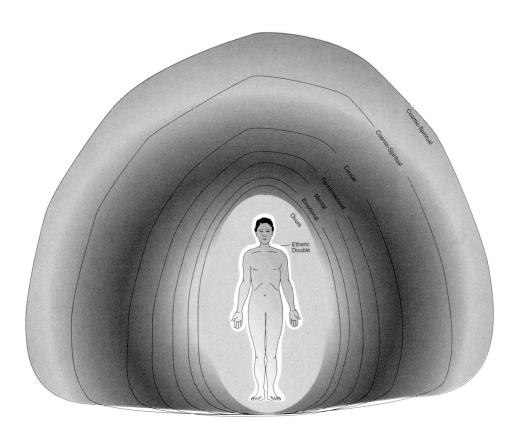

CHAKRA LOCATIONS

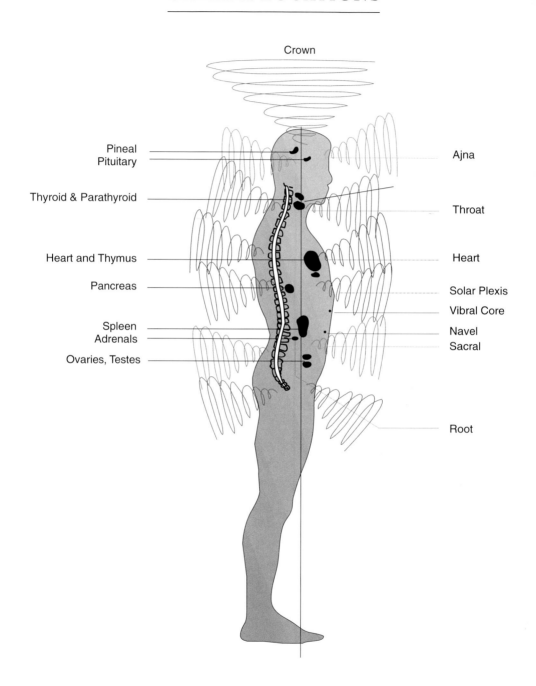

Crown

Pineal
Pituitary

Ajna

Thyroid & Parathyroid

Throat

Heart and Thymus

Heart

Pancreas

Solar Plexis

Vibral Core

Spleen
Adrenals

Navel
Sacral

Ovaries, Testes

Root

ENERGY SPIRAL

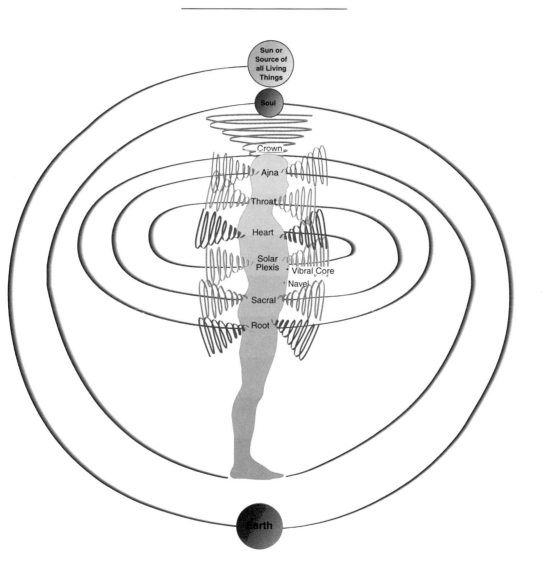

EGG MEDITATION

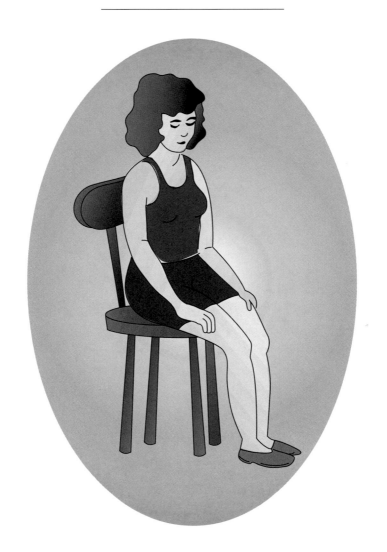

3-POINT MEDITATION

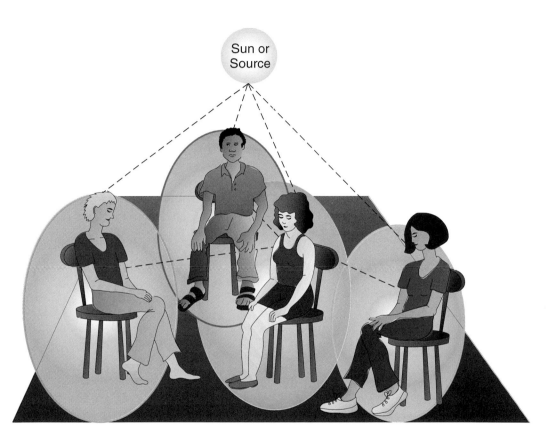

RAINBOW DISK

Step 1

Step 2

Step 3

6

Centering

"Centering" yourself, in essence, means to shift your consciousness from the instability of everyday life to the quiet calm of your own spiritual core. In the center of your inner being lies a peace and stability that cannot be shaken by events outside of you. As your consciousness becomes ever more founded upon this inner spiritual base, you become more tranquil, emotionally stable, and powerful in understated and balanced ways.

Typically, our awareness is subject to the volatile world of everyday cares and concerns. Our physical, emotional, and psychological condition is predicated on events that take place outside of us—on whether or not we had a good day at work, for example, or how other people treat us. As people and events change, the quality of your life rises and falls. The more attached you are to the events and the behavior of others, the more reactive and unstable you become.

To center yourself, by contrast, means to anchor your awareness in the spiritual roots of your life. To be centered in your spiritual roots means to shift your consciousness from life's daily tumult to the center of your soul, the place within you that continually draws life energy from its universal source. Here, at your vital center, is the place from which your life truly springs.

Life itself is energy, and the source of energy is the One, the Great Spirit, the Tao. To attune your consciousness to the center of being is to align yourself with the will of the universe and to be nourished by its never-ending flow of life energy. (I will offer several meditations to help you achieve a centered state shortly.)

The effects of such a shift in awareness are transformative in every respect. Rather than being tossed around by the external travails of the ephemeral world, you are now grounded in the unchanging world of universal life force. Hence, you are at peace. The level of physical tension in your body drops precipitously. Scientific research has shown that people in meditation exhibit high degrees of alertness, concentration, and synchronicity between the left and right hemispheres of the brain. Heart rate and breathing patterns slow, blood pressure stabilizes, and skin conductivity decreases, a sign that circulation has improved. Dolores Krieger conducted a pilot study on practitioners of healing touch and found that they also achieved this same meditative state and thus experienced many of the same biological changes that sitting meditators undergo.

Various cultures and religious traditions have developed far-reaching understandings of what it truly means to be centered. The entire Japanese culture is founded upon the ethic that all behavior should flow from the vital center of being, or what the Japanese call *hara*. All the Japanese martial and cultural arts—from judo to painting to flower arranging to music—are meant to be expressions of the vital center. To be centered, say Japanese and Chinese philosophers, is to reconcile heaven and earth.

Perhaps for this reason, centering makes you acutely aware of yourself as a whole human being—that is, you become aware of your physical body, your emotions, and your spiritual consciousness as an integrated totality. Centering is a meditative act and an act of integration and harmony.

Virtually all traditional philosophy has recognized that we humans are being pulled constantly by the two archetypal extremes within our consciousness—the instinctual world of the physical senses and physical desires, and the intellectual and spiritual realms of ethics and ideals. These two archetypes cannot be balanced or harmonized by any intellectual or mental act. Indeed, as every adult knows, to settle this existential conflict through an activity of the mind is to settle it in favor of the mind, and thus to deny the needs of the body. Traditional peoples have maintained that the only way the two extremes can be reconciled and brought into harmony is to shift one's consciousness to the center of being, the vital center, which is beyond mind, concepts, and the changing standards of right and wrong. Here, in the spiritual center, lies the reconciliation of all opposites within life.

Carl Jung concurred with this view. In *Alchemical Studies,* he points out that the "center is compared to paradise and its four rivers." The four rivers connote the four directions of the earth, or the relative world. The place where the rivers converge and are joined, the center, is the place where the four cardinal directions are all reconciled and made one. "Nothing is more like God than the centre," writes Jung, "for it occupies no space, and cannot be grasped, seen or measured. Such too, is the nature of God and spirits." Indeed, Jung, like the great alchemists before him, most notably Paracelsus, maintained that meditation and the shifting of consciousness to the center of being brings about the perception of the invisible or spiritual world.

Jung quotes Gerard Dorn and his book on alchemy, *Theatrum Chemicum,* in which Dorn states that "all things which likewise fill no place because they lack body, as is the case with all spirits, can be comprehended in the centre, for both are incomprehensible. As therefore there is no end of the centre, no pen can rightly describe its power and the infinite abyss of its mysteries."

Perhaps because the center is the place of such "infinite mysteries," we recognize that from here springs all that is sacred into the material world. Thus, to center oneself means to approach the sacred or divine within.

Centering, therefore, is a meditative act that transforms you physically, psychologically, and spiritually. The practitioner of healing touch begins a session by centering herself. In this way, she places herself in right relationship with the universal energy and thus attains the right standpoint for participating in the flow of that energy.

This is the mental framework that the practitioner of healing touch attempts to achieve. When you are centered, you have no judgments about the person you are working with, nor do you have any attachments to outcome. You are not the source of the healing. You are not in control of what takes place. The energy flows from the divine source, through you, and to the recipient of healing touch. You, as a practitioner of healing touch, submit yourself as an instrument of that divine source. Whatever outcome occurs for the client is between the creator of the universe and the recipient. In a way, you, as the practitioner, are a witness to the outcome.

Elisabeth Kübler-Ross, M.D., in her essay "The Four Pillars of Healing," refers to the healer as a channel, or as she puts it "a conduit of a healing entity or force." Healers, shamans, and medicine men or women have referred to this same healing energy as Yahweh, Great Spirit, God, the Christed Energy, or the Higher Self. However one refers to it, it is this divine energy that creates the healing, regardless of the healer's technique. Twylah Nitsch, my Seneca teacher, also points out that the healer not only opens as a channel for the Great Mystery, but also must come from a place of faith and gratitude. No healing can occur without faith and gratitude.

As Dr. Kübler-Ross points out, healers do not heal. The very title "healer" is a bit of a misnomer, because the true healer is the Great Healer. The practitioner is more a facilitator, a participant, and a witness. He or she is not the source of healing.

This is often a difficult fact to recognize because, as a compassionate human being, you want to help others. Indeed, one of your primary motivations for doing healing touch is to be of service. Also, there is the added pressure that we all feel to prove that the practice works, that this is not a fringe or charlatan practice but a highly effective form of treatment. Yet, the essence of the practice is to surrender all control of outcome because the energy that you help to transmit will be utilized by the recipient's body however the body needs the life force.

In explaining the mysterious nature of healing, Dolores Krieger, a pioneer of healing touch, showed in her essay "The Timeless Concept of Healing" why a practitioner must ultimately surrender to larger forces that control the healing process. As healers, we cannot know every level of what the patient needs for complete healing. Dr. Krieger points out that just on a physiological level, the myriad biological functions are "exquisitely synchronized." When we add the emotional levels of healing, it becomes even more complicated. Therefore, when we approach our patients, part of our prayer must be, "Thy will be done." We have faith that the incredible human and divine energies come together to create the exact transformation for healing that is needed.

True healers have always understood their humble, yet essential role in the healing process. Even the Father of Medicine, Hippocrates, understood his position in the face of the mysteries that healing invokes. For all of his wisdom and knowledge, which at the time towered above all others, Hippocrates recognized that divine powers ultimately decided the final fate of every illness. As he said some 2,500 years ago, "The healing art involves a weaving of a knowledge of the gods into the texture of the physician's mind. The Art is held in honor by the gods, in its relations not only to bodily mishaps but to bodily conditions generally. For it is not by individual cleverness that a physician is effective. Although he has his hands on many aspects of an ailment, it may still happen that the cure comes about quite spontaneously. Of course whatever contributions the healing art is able to make should be accepted from it. But the path of wisdom in the Art lies in making final acknowledgment to Those Very Ones."

Thus, the most important attitudes that the practitioner must maintain toward a client, as well as toward himself or herself, are compassion, love, honesty (especially with himself or herself), and humility. This is how the practitioner of healing touch confronts the sacred drama that he or she is witness to and assists.

It is also why it is so important to begin every session of healing touch by centering yourself. By centering yourself in your own spiritual roots, you are not so easily distracted by anyone's emotions or desires, or even by the explicit needs of the client. Rather, you are respectful of the client and his or her relationship with the Creator. Once you are centered, you come into communion with the source of the energy that truly heals. Then, whatever that energy desires to happen will happen, effortlessly.

Being Present and Grounded to Be the Clearest Channel

Once you have centered yourself, of course, you must firmly maintain your center through the course of your healing touch session. To do that you must sustain your concentration and be fully present with your client. You can't suddenly drift off in your mind and begin to think about the many demands in your own life. Such wandering off will affect the flow of energy that is traveling through you to your client and thus make the session less effective. Also, the more you wander, the more you diminish the sense of the sacred. The client's awareness of the sacred is part of what allows him or her to accept the life energy that's being offered. The best way for you to sincerely invoke the sacred is through your own centeredness and concentration. Most forms of ceremony ring false and ultimately cast you in the wrong light. You are a professional practitioner who must maintain his or her professional standpoint. Yet, you are dealing with powers far beyond your comprehension, or mine, and therefore must be respectful of the true source of the healing energy that you transmit. As I pointed out earlier, the best and perhaps only way to strike the right balance between your earthly role and your heavenly

ideals is to remain centered and focused. In the center, all paradoxes are reconciled, and the sense of the sacred is invoked without your doing anything.

In order to keep myself focused and centered, I do a visualization before the session and recite a prayer during it. Therefore,
before you conduct your healing touch session, do the following:

First, place your feet firmly on the floor, about shoulder-width
apart. Feel the energy in your legs and feet anchor itself in the floor.
Visualize it going deeply into the earth so that the earth holds you
in its embrace. Feel yourself being supported by the earth and nourished by the energy that flows upward from the Great Mother. At
the same time, feel the upper levels of your own energy reach up
into the heavens, just as the limbs of a tree reach into the sky. Feel
the love of the heavens rain down on the limbs of your field and
surround and envelop you. See the love and energy come up from
the earth and mingle with that of the heavens. Visualize that energy
channeling itself into your entire body and down into your arms
and hands. See it flow from your hands. You now have the healing
energy to channel to your client.

Before I turn to my client, however, I recite a prayer. I say this
prayer over and over again throughout the healing session to remain focused on the work. I share this prayer with you as a basis for
creating your own prayer, or for adopting it yourself. The prayer is
as follows:

"Father, Mother, God, I place myself and this patient in your
Holy Light for the Highest Good of all. I ask that You work through
me to bring healing to this patient. From Thee, through me, to this
patient. I ask that Thy Will be done, and I am grateful for this
healing."

If you create your own prayer, I encourage you to include the
phrases "for the Highest Good of all," "Thy Will be done," and a
phrase of gratitude for the healing that is taking place. These
phrases assist you in your efforts to surrender the outcome to the
higher power or Tao. Remember, surrender is not giving up, but
rather giving over control and outcome to the Great Mystery that is

the true healer. By reciting this prayer, you are acknowledging your faith in the Creator and its power to heal. You are also offering yourself as a participant and a servant in that process.

Finally, as you do your energy work on your client, visualize the darkness, boulders, and blockages that are being released from your client's field as being absorbed into the light and love of the heavens, or ethers. The earth takes these energetic blockages, stones, and old patterns and dissolves them into the soil, transforming them into elements that support life and renewed growth.

Be sure to do the egg meditation, given below, before you begin to work with your client. This will protect you from the energetic imbalances and illnesses your client may be suffering from.

Before You Proceed, Know How You Feel

Your centering and grounding meditations will put you in touch with your physical body and your emotions. You'll know how you feel and, if you allow your emotions to fully surface, you will know why you have such feelings. Do not resist or repress such emotions, or the events that surround them, but rather embrace and honor these feelings. No matter what surfaces, whether it is anger, shame, humiliation, or conflict, try to examine the feelings and have compassion for yourself. Such emotions—and the events that triggered them—are part of what it means to be human. With continued meditation, you will be able to integrate these and other feelings. You will be able to see the courage you had to have to go through such events. In time, you will be able to honor yourself in ways that perhaps you cannot do now. You will also become more proficient at opening your heart and entering into a consciousness of nonjudgment and acceptance.

However, if you cannot reconcile these emotions in the moment, or create peace within yourself, you are better off avoiding the day's healing touch sessions.

Powerful emotions, especially anger or hatred, are inappropriate to a healing touch session. There is a good chance that you will transmit such vibrations to your client. Or you may not be able to maintain your concentration and groundedness to protect yourself from your client's energy or illness. You are better off avoiding the whole interaction and postponing it to another day. In the meantime, work on yourself. Remember what I said in chapter 1: The greatest demands made on a practitioner of healing touch are those the practitioner makes of himself or herself. He or she must become more open-hearted, loving, compassionate, clear, and less attached to outcome. The practitioner must become more centered in the spiritual roots of his or her being, and thus clearer about who he or she is, who the client is, and who the healer is.

Being Centered Means Respecting Your Limits

As a practitioner of healing touch, you are performing an invaluable service to your client, to the healing arts, and to the world at large. You are providing your client with an enormous boost of healing energy, energy that is essential for the client's restoration and recovery. By offering this service, you are giving people a new tool to restore health, as well as a new approach to understanding, health, illness, and, indeed, life itself. Finally, you are serving as an instrument of love and healing, something in very short supply in our world today.

Yet, despite this incredibly important role, many practitioners of healing touch nevertheless feel they must be more, and in the process make the mistake of overstepping their own boundaries, and the client's. You must always keep in mind the scope of your practice in order to be effective in your job as a healer. Always remember that your central function is to serve as a conduit for healing energy. You promote the flow of the life force in other people. Whatever your client does with that energy is between him or her and God. The person already knows what he or she needs to be healed, though this knowledge may not be conscious. Nevertheless, you must release the client into the hands of the Universal Healer in order to do the most good. You are not responsible for the client's recovery, any more than you are responsible for the client's disharmony or disease. You are assisting the client in her or his journey through life and, specifically, in her or his attempts to get well. You are the helper, the server, the practitioner of a powerful healing tool. You do not have to diagnose or provide insight into the person's past disharmonies. You do not have to be a psychotherapist, or a medical doctor, or a nurse, if these are not your professions.

People will want you to be more at times. Indeed, you will be tempted to be more, in part because the practice requires so much faith, especially in the beginning when you lack experience and haven't seen the incredible effects you can have on people just by doing this seemingly simple job. This lack of experience may tempt you to fill the knowledge gap with promises or speculation. Resist these temptations with all your strength. Instead, become both a practitioner and an investigator of this practice. See for yourself what it can do. Fill up your life and your practice with real experience. Really come to know how the practice affects other people, how it changes lives and restores health. When you do this, your words will be based on what is true and real, rather than on what you think or have read. The practice works, but you must experience it working before you know in your heart that it works. Let yourself have that experience.

Follow these three rules and you will be safe in all situations:

1. Be honest with yourself; when you don't know something, admit it to yourself. Embracing your humanness is one of the most wonderful and transformative experiences you will ever have. The more you can do this simple act, the more you stand in the light of truth, the greater your own transformation, and the more powerful you become.

2. Be honest with your client; don't be trapped into inflating your role, or your knowledge, or your ego, even if it means making

the client uncomfortable temporarily. People naturally want reassurance, and you will want to give it. But sometimes that mutual desire can lure you into implying things, or promising things, that you cannot be certain of. It is better to say "I don't know" than to offer people promises that later turn out to be false or illusory. You are centered and powerful whenever you speak the truth, even if the truth is merely admitting your limitations.

3.   Respect yourself. You are taking up a role that, in other cultures and traditions, was among the most revered and honored functions in human society. Today, all practitioners of the holistic healing arts are pioneers, offering people powerful tools for establishing health. We are bringing back to the modern world the keys to health that temporarily have been forgotten. Slowly, but inexorably, holistic healing is being restored to the place of honor that was once the natural place for herbalists, acupuncturists, practitioners of Chinese medicine, Ayurveda, bodyworkers, shamans, and practitioners of healing touch. As long as you are clear about your practice and what you do, you are performing an essential service that is not being duplicated by any other profession. You belong in the healing arts. And you do not have to be any more than what you are. As you gain experience in this practice, you will learn firsthand that that is quite enough.

Meditations for Centering

MEDITATION #1

Sit in a chair with your back straight and your feet flat on the floor, hands resting on your knees. Relax. Take in a deep breath and begin an easy exhale, making an "aaahhh" sound with your voice box. After a few seconds (two or three), suspend the noise and the exhale without closing the throat. The throat should feel open as it did when you made the "aaahhh" sound. After a few seconds let the breath exhale. Repeat this two more times. You should notice by the third time that you are able to hold your breath longer. When you open your eyes the room should appear brighter. You are centered and probably in an alpha brain wave state.

MEDITATION #2: THE EGG MEDITATION

1. Sit in a comfortable chair with your feet flat on the floor, hands on your knees.
2. Take a few deep even breaths and then begin to breathe rhythmically. Concentrate on your breath. Watch the breath.
3. Meanwhile, let go of all thoughts. If any thought enters your mind, watch it float into and out of your consciousness. Feel your consciousness enter more deeply into your body.
4. Picture yourself enclosed in an egg-shaped bubble that surrounds you at a distance of about an arm's length. Feel the outer edge as kind of a strong, semipermeable membrane, something like a Plexiglas shield, that allows only positive, loving energy to escape your inner being and the bubble; the bubble only allows such loving, supportive, and positive energy to enter the bubble and embrace you, as well.
5. Balance the front and the back of the egg or bubble so that the energy feels equal on all sides. This balances the output of energy between the front and back chakras.
6. Maintain a steady, slow, rhythmic breath, noting any places in your body where you are holding tension. Breathe into that tension and release it.
7. Notice your posture. Maintain your centeredness and an erect posture with your breath.
8. See the protective energetic shield as a force of invulnerable love. It is designed to protect you, while it allows you to help others.

This meditation is not designed to place boundaries between you and your client, or between you and the world. Rather, it is designed to maintain the integrity of your own energy field, to close any leaks, and to allow you to focus the healing energy that you are channeling in your work. The egg meditation is designed to create a powerful sphere around you so that you will be protected from your client's energetic imbalances, disharmonies, and any illnesses the client may be suffering from. This bubble is composed of your loving energy, and thus vibrates at a rate that is not conducive to your client's disharmony or imbalance. Anything that your client sheds or releases during the session, therefore, will not be able to attach itself to you.

MEDITATION #3

In his book *Awaken Healing Energy Through the Tao,* Korean healer and teacher Mantah Chia provides a meditation that teaches us to circulate the Qi throughout the body. This meditation helps each of us, as practitioners, restore our own health and maintain balance and harmony. Once again, the responsibility of the practitioner—especially one who works with the transmission of energy—is to keep his or her own field clean and health strong.

Sit in a quiet, peaceful room, on a comfortable chair, with your back straight and your feet flat on the floor. Rub your hands, feet, arms, and legs with your hands. Rotate your neck. Place your hands in your lap with both palms up, your right hand resting on top of your left. Your eyes can be open or closed, though closing them will make it easier to visualize during the meditation. Then perform the following steps:

1. Look down into your body and smile down the front line of the upper part of your body. Smile into your eyes; smile to your face, neck, throat, heart, blood and circulatory system, lungs, kidneys, adrenals, liver, pancreas, and spleen.
2. Now smile down the mid-line of your digestive tract. Smile to your esophagus and stomach. Swallow your saliva and let it

carry the smile down into those organs. Smile down into your small intestine, down into your large intestine, rectum, and anus. Continue to swallow saliva and visualize it carrying your smile downward through your entire digestive tract.

3. Focus on the back of your body. Send your smile down the spine, vertebra by vertebra.
4. Release your jaws and touch the tongue to the palate.
5. Complete the meditation by collecting the energy at the navel. Spiral the energy inside the navel one and a half inches deep. Women should spiral the energy thirty-six times counterclockwise and twenty-four times clockwise. Men should spiral the energy in the opposite direction—thirty-six times clockwise and twenty-four times counterclockwise.

This inner smile will have profound changes on your life if done every day, as it begins to repattern the energy flow through your entire body.

The following meditation is designed to help you, the healer, center and clear your own energy.

EXERCISE #4—CENTERING AND CLEARING

1. Take some deep breaths, relaxing your mind, letting go of all thoughts and words. Feel the relaxed rhythm of your breath.
2. Picture a small globe of light that is your soul about six inches above your head. Above that, picture a larger globe of light that is the sun or the source of all living things (The Light of Love).
3. Slowly visualize a beam of light full of all colors of the rainbow from the source through your soul into your crown. Feel the crown chakra take the color that it needs to expand this area. Release what is no longer useful there into the Light of Love.
4. Drop the rainbow light into the brow of the third eye. Feel the color that is needed expand from the rainbow and be released

into the chakra. Feel the area expand and release what it no longer needs into the Light of Love.

5. Let the rainbow light descend into the throat chakra, filling it with light, expanding and releasing.
6. Fill the heart space, expanding and releasing.
7. Visualize the light moving into the solar plexus, expanding and releasing.
8. Next, visualize the energy moving down into the sacral chakra, expanding and releasing.
9. Now fill the root chakra with this light, expanding and releasing.
10. Split the light, seeing it travel down both legs, exiting through the arches in the feet, going deeply into the earth.
11. Feel the rainbow of colors fill you. Feel the peace and balance. Feel the connection with the source as you ground to the earth.
12. When you are ready and it feels right, open your eyes and let your light shine.

All of these techniques will center you in your spiritual roots. They will also help to balance your energetic field, will open the tube down the center of the field to allow the free flow of energy through the body, and ultimately will help to heal you.

Now, let's turn our attention to yet another layer of helping others—specifically, using the hands to heal.

7

Assessing the Energy Field

When I begin to work with a person, I spend time trying to understand the client's specific issues. I begin by asking the person to fill out an intake questionnaire that describes his or her current symptoms and conditions (see appendix 1). The questionnaire requests information on current health complaints, if any; health history; any herbs or medication being taken; and the person's reasons for seeing me. If the person is not seeing a physician or some other health professional at the time he or she comes to me, I recommend one or another whom I know or whose work I respect. Nothing I do is meant to replace the work of a medical doctor or other appropriate health care professionals. Healing touch is meant to complement the work of a physician, not to compete with it. This is especially important if the person is suffering from a serious illness.

Once the questionnaire has been filled out, I discuss any health, psychological, or interpersonal disharmonies he or she may be experiencing as part of an initial interview. I want to get to know the person I'll be working with in such an intimate and important way. The discussion can involve any aspect of a person's life that is a source of stress or disharmony, ranging from a personal health issue to a marital or financial problem. In addition to getting to know the person, I also try to figure out where in the field the person's problems may be rooted. As I listen to and observe him or her, I try to discern which chakras or areas within the field may be involved in the person's disharmony and where I should begin working.

Once I have some insight into the problem, I assess the energy field. I do this for all my clients, even those whom I have been seeing regularly for some time. I begin by having the person sit on a stool, so that all sides of the field and body are exposed. (If you do not have such a stool, have the person sit in a straight-backed chair so that the chair's back is to his or her immediate left. This will allow you to move your hands through the front and back of the person's field.) Also, I ask my client to take off his or her shoes before I start the session. This allows me to determine whether or not the energy is flowing freely from the feet when I assess that part of the field. I stand behind the seated person, center myself, and as I do, I stand with my left hand raised above my head, with the palm of my hand facing the sky. My right arm is down at my side, slightly away from my body, with the palm facing downward toward the earth (see the photograph 3 on page 225). Now I am receiving the life force from the two poles of life, so to speak, heaven and earth. While in this position, I am saying my prayer.

When I feel deeply centered, I bring my hands together and feel the spongy ball (described in chapter 3)—soft, fluffy, and resilient—between my hands. It's about the size of a basketball, perhaps a little smaller. I feel the ball in front of me at the level of my vibral core. I then move the ball in my hands toward the person's vibral core, at his back, visualizing the connection of my vibral core to the patient through the energy ball. Then I move to my patient's right side and place my hands about a foot over his head. I dissolve the energy ball into his field and "see" it enrich his field with life force. Slowly, I allow my hands to come apart and simultaneously move down the front and back of the patient's field, all the while assessing his energy. My hands are anywhere from six to eighteen inches from the person's body. Meanwhile, I am reciting my prayer to remain centered and empty of distracting thoughts.

"Seeing" and "Listening" with Your Touch

I assess the field with my hands, but in effect I am touching the field with my entire being. I am so attuned to the energy that I am feeling it with a type of perception that is the synthesis of all my physical perceptions and yet is beyond my physical perceptions. It's as if my physical perceptions and those of my higher self all combine to form a singular intelligence, a unified perception, that goes just beyond my everyday senses. Thus, as I touch the field, I am "listening" to it with my hands; I am "seeing" it with my fingers; I am sensing something that might be thought of as smell or taste but goes beyond these as well.

As I conduct my assessment, I move my hands downward from the top of the client's head and down the front and back of the body. I run my hands gently over the field in the area of the heart (right hand) and the back of the lungs (left hand), over the stomach and kidneys, over the lower intestinal tract and lumbar area of the spine, over the front and back of the legs, and down to the feet. Meanwhile, I note any imbalance or deviation from that resilient ball of "cotton candy." I feel how resilient and closed the field feels in most places, as if there is an egg-shaped energy with a specific boundary area. As I move my hands farther along the periphery of the field, I may begin to perceive aberrations.

Perceiving Changes in Temperature and Density

The most common sensation is a very subtle resilience, which dominates most people's fields, or what I referred to in chapter 2 as "cotton candy." Changes in temperature are also common. Some places may feel cool, others cold; some places in the field are warm, and occasionally I encounter significant heat.

In general, you typically do not feel a change in temperature when going over the client's field. However, whenever you do notice a decline in temperature—a relatively cool or cold spot—it can often mean a decrease in energy and may appear over places where there is little life force. Those energy dips may indicate that that part of the body was wounded long ago, causing a diminished flow of blood, lymph, and life force to that area and creating the conditions for a disharmony of some kind. The person may not experience the underlying conditions until the disharmony reaches an acute phase, but long before the physical body experiences the disorder, the underlying energetic causes of disharmony were already present.

Low back injuries are a good example of this phenomenon. It is quite common for people to experience a low back injury simply by bending down and picking up a newspaper—hardly a strenuous task. In fact, the conditions for the injury were there within the back muscles and vertebrae for a long time—sometimes for more than a decade—before these underlying conditions suddenly went from a latent or dormant phase to an acute phase disorder. Picking up the newspaper was simply the proverbial "straw" that served only as the catalyst of the injury. The energy within the back becomes increasingly imbalanced—too much energy in some places, too little in others—until the extremes cause an acute imbalance in the muscles of the back, manifesting as excessive contraction among certain muscles and excessive weakness in others. The spinal vertebrae are kept in alignment by muscle tension that is essentially equal on the left and right sides of the spine. However, muscles on one side usually become too contracted and lose their flexibility; they can no longer expand and contract within their normal ranges. Other muscles become excessively weak and thus can no longer support the vertebrae or other muscles, meaning that one side of the back muscles is pulling harder than the other side. Eventually, the smallest action—such as picking up a newspaper—can cause the contracted muscles to go into spasm and in the process pull the vertebrae to one side of the back. On the other side, the weak muscles give way, allowing the spine to curve unnaturally in the direction of the contracted muscles. This causes the spine to force the vertebrae to pinch nerves and is perceived as an acute injury. Once the condition reaches an acute phase, the area becomes inflamed and hot. Heat is often a sign of increased circulation, inflammation, and sometimes fever—all symptoms of the acute phase.

Stones and Boulders: The Blockages that Bind

To understand the nature of energetic blockages, you must recognize that energy is constantly moving through the field in great channels, like rushing rivers. As long as the energy is circulating through the field and physical body, there is an abundance of life force flowing to organs, tissues, and cells, and thus there is health and harmony within the entire system. Disharmony arises when the energy is blocked. Your job, as a practitioner of healing touch, is to remove those blockages and to send additional life force to areas that have been deprived of energy.

When a river is blocked with a stone or debris, water swirls around the blockage, creating eddies. Also, in front of the stone is an overabundance of water—it builds up and swells high on the rock—while at the other side of the stone the water is low. The side of the stone that faces the oncoming energy is therefore excessive in energy, while the side of the stone that is opposite is deficient. It's the same in the energetic field of the human body. Blockages exist like the stones, or boulders, that create eddies in some areas, excesses in others, and deficiencies in still others. In fact, blockages almost always create excess energy in the foreground and deficiencies in the lee. Boulders tie up life force, or bind it, thus blocking it from flowing abundantly to other areas of the field and body. An example is Wendy, the person I spoke about in chapter 2, who is overcoming MS. Wendy experienced blockages behind the neck, and a deficiency of energy in the limbs.

Deficiencies in the field can be perceived as the absence of energy, and sometimes as a hole, or what I refer to as a leak. Holes or leaks arise not just from blockages elsewhere in the field but also from traumas experienced early in life that inflicted wounds on the energetic body.

Holes in the Field: The Physical Locations of Guilt and Shame

Holes or leaks are energetic patterns within the field that allow energy to escape, causing the person to experience a sudden change in emotions (usually bringing on negative emotions), a loss of energy, and a loss of his or her personal integrity. A common symptom of a leak is a negative emotional pattern that is consistent but usually irrational. Leaks trigger feelings of guilt, shame, anger, low self-esteem, and personal failure.

Leaks in the field, and their corresponding emotional patterns, are established in childhood, when parents or guardians teach children how to react to difficult situations that may involve personal responsibility. They are also caused by physical or psychological abuse. Such abuse injures the field literally, causing a tear or rip or hole. We must remember that verbal or physical abuse is an energetic and vibrational act as well as a physical act. A parent need not strike a child to make the child feel injured; the injury can be accomplished just as effectively—and sometimes even more permanently—with a word or a set of words, especially if those words are shouted in anger or rage. Sometimes, that is the very reason the words are said in the first place, though few people would admit it: They are meant to "wound." The effects of such verbal or vibrational attacks on the field are analogous to striking your arm with your fist. If you strike your arm for a certain amount of time, you will cause the capillaries to be broken and your arm will turn black and blue; if you persist, you will eventually break the skin; and if you persist still longer, you will break the bone. Energetic attacks on one's field are done with the emotional vibration and the intent that is embedded in words and attitudes. This vibration causes an actual wound in the energy field, just as striking your arm causes a physical wound in your flesh. An emotional or psychological wound will leak life energy from the child's—and later the adult's—field until it is healed.

Every human being counts on his or her field to give a clear sense of self, of boundaries, that describes the limits of his or her responsibility in any given situation. To know one's limits is to have control over one's life. When a child's field has a hole in it (or numerous holes, for that matter), the child does not learn a healthy sense of boundaries and has no clear or realistic understanding of personal responsibility. Without such boundaries, the life energy is drawn out of the child's field, the sense of self is weakened, and the child is susceptible to being unhealthfully influenced by other people's values, identities, needs, and desires. The child or adult may come to identify so thoroughly with another human being that he or she adopts that other person's desires as if they were his or her own, living only to please another human being. The child cannot feel any sense of self-worth unless everyone else in his life, including his family members and other key people, are happy and satisfied. This, of course, means that the child can never be happy or centered. He will always try to please others because his life force is constantly extending to and overlapping with others, thus causing him to identify too much with the needs of others. This emotional and energetic pattern determines a child's beliefs about himself, his family, and the world. It affects how a child interprets experience and whether or not he can utilize his own strengths in certain situations.

Even when a child reaches adulthood, he still experiences guilt or shame or anguish whenever he confronts similar situations as those that created the initial hole and energy leak. Once again, he loses his sense of self, of perspective, of boundaries, even of self-protection. In a sense, he doesn't see reality; instead, he feels his pain, or rather, he reexperiences an old, ongoing, and ever-repeating pain. It's the same old drama: Someone close to him isn't happy; he feels he is to blame for that person's pain, so he himself cannot be happy. Thus, he experiences a loss of energy, of integrity, and all the same old feelings of guilt, shame, anger, and injustice. At bottom, he feels he isn't worthy of love or life, especially self-love. In order to compensate for such feelings, he often finds himself doing more than what is actually asked of him, which results in a tremendous expenditure of energy. The resulting praise is often sufficient reward—at least for a time—and can drive a person to high degrees of self-denial. Such a person becomes increasingly self-deprecating. Eventually, his needs begin to surface, however, but because he was trained—and maintained his own training—to deny himself, the result is often anger and even bitterness. This sets up a pattern of ongoing leaks.

To some extent, a hole in the field is always leaking a relatively small amount of energy, even in those situations when the person is not made to feel inferior or shameful. Leaks will continually drain energy, which is why the person who has such leaks closed—even for a short period of time—experiences a sudden increase in energy and overall vitality. This is why I say that closing leaks is one of the most important functions in healing touch.

Guilt: The Wound that Stays Alive by Keeping You Blind to Its Existence

Guilt and shame are the most common emotions to surface whenever leaks in the field are exposed. Guilt makes you feel that you should have done something that you didn't, or that you shouldn't have done something that you did. The implicit belief that gives rise to guilt is that you could have been more than you were, which is a delusion. You cannot be more than you are at any given moment. Each situation arises and you meet it with the physical, psychological, and spiritual resources you have available in that moment. You can be nothing more, nor anything less.

To better understand guilt, we must see the difference between guilt and remorse. Guilt is a chronic feeling, an unhealed wound, that reminds us that we need to be healed. Remorse, on the other hand, is the feeling of deep sorrow for having hurt someone. Deeply felt remorse leads to change. Guilt, conversely, tends to maintain its own patterns. This is the irony of guilt, because you would think that because guilt is so unpleasant, it would prevent us from repeating the same pattern, but it doesn't work that way. *Guilt actually stops us from examining our pain.* Guilt gives rise to a pain that is inarticulate, imprecise, and opaque. Very often, we're not sure why we feel guilty; all we know is that we do. But the underlying belief below the pain is that, somehow, we should have been a different person from the person we were.

Guilt is a wound in the field that leaks energy. Certain energetic patterns in the field and in the person's behavior and thinking may keep that wound from healing. As a consequence, each time one meets a situation that resembles the one that caused the original wound, these same feelings occur.

Guilt and shame, in a subtle yet powerful way, cause all of us to lose our sense of integrity, self-protection, and centeredness. Whoever the person is who has made you feel guilty has managed to open one of these leaky places. Once that happens, you give yourself over to the person's judgment of you, as if he or she had the greater hold on truth. Your own personal integrity has broken down; you feel weaker, more unsure, energetically ill-defined, as if you no longer have a clear sense of who you are, where you begin, and where you end. This loss of clarity is due to the breakdown of your own energetic boundary, a boundary that protects you, identifies you, encloses you within it, and gives you a feeling of integrity, wholeness, and strength.

Looking for the Clues to Guide the Course of Healing

Once I have located an imbalance in the field—no matter what type it is—I note the area, its nearest chakra, and its correspondence to the body. I look for clues that will reveal the source or sources of the imbalance. If the imbalance is over the heart area, for example, I note the possibility of a disharmony in the heart chakra, the possibility of an emotional issue, and perhaps some form of heart disease. If it is over the lower abdomen, I wonder about the health of the large intestine or sex organs; if it is over the solar plexus, I wonder about the liver (particularly if the imbalance is on the right side of the body), or the spleen/pancreas (if it is over the left), or the stomach (if it is directly in the center). An imbalance over the solar plexus, or just below it, might also suggest that the stomach and small intestine are in distress.

I also keep in mind the spiral of energy, which reveals how energy moves through and nourishes the chakras. As you will recall from chapter 4, the order in which the life force moves through the chakras is from the fourth chakra to the third, then to the fifth, to the second, to the sixth, to the first, and then to the seventh. Headaches (a sixth chakra disorder) may be caused by a first or second chakra imbalance. Sore throats (a fifth chakra disorder) may be caused by a third or second chakra imbalance. Whenever I encounter a known symptom, I look for the corresponding chakra imbalance. I also examine the chakras directly above and below the disorder. I am looking for any evidence of excessive or deficient energy that may cause an imbalance in its neighboring chakra. This is particularly true if the condition is chronic and standard medical treatment has been unable to cure it.

Posture: A Window into Imbalance

Both the field and the physical body maintain a dynamic equilibrium. An excess in one place typically creates a deficiency in another. The two extremes work in tandem, often creating visible distortions in the physical body. Posture is an outstanding example of this. The posture will express clearly where excesses and deficiencies lie. When you see a person with a large, expanded upper back and a concave chest, this type of posture creates a dis-

tinct S-shaped curve in the body when looked at from the right
side, with the shoulder area curved back and the stomach curved
in. The upper back seems bigger and fleshier; the chest seems
smaller and retracted; the stomach area is pushed forward. Such a
posture prevents deep breathing, which means that the breath is
most active in the upper lung area and least active in the lower.
This means that the upper part of the lungs is expanded and excessive in energy—they are the part doing the most breathing—
while the lower lobes of the lung are contracted and deficient of
energy. There are probably large blockages of energy over the
neck and back, preventing the life force from going deeply into
the lungs. Without sufficient life force, the lower part of the
lungs will contract, and then atrophy, and eventually manifest a
symptom.

Shallow breathing forces the heart to work harder to pump
sufficient oxygen to cells; this causes the heart to beat more rapidly.
In all likelihood, the heart is tired and overworked, which means
that despite its rapid beating—or rather, because of it—the heart is
deficient. The small intestine, which is responsible for absorption of
nutrients, is probably contracted, meaning that the organ itself has
narrowed. The villi, which are fingerlike projections in the organ
that absorb nutrients, are coated with bacteria and enmeshed with
each other, preventing them from optimally absorbing nutrition.
The large intestine, responsible for absorption of water and elimination of waste, is expanded physically and becomes sluggish in its
function. The organ is swollen, has lost muscle tone, and can eventually suffer from diverticulosis. The large intestine also lacks life
force, or is deficient of energy. Both of these symptoms are revealed
by the contraction in the upper stomach area and the swollen abdomen. In short, the person suffers from any of a variety of heart,
lung, and digestive disorders, including either constipation or diarrhea. This type of posture invariably causes problems in the second
chakra (lower abdomen), the third (solar plexus), the fourth
(heart), and the fifth (throat).

Many middle-aged men often present distended stomachs, especially in the area of the solar plexus (third chakra), while the kidney area (second chakra) is curved inward, toward the front of the body. The posture looks like a bow—or one long outward curve from the face to the bottom of the torso. The person does not have to be terribly overweight: The distention and swelling of the stomach varies widely depending on the person and his relative imbalance. Nevertheless, when viewed from the side, the person seems to be all front and no back. This stature is particularly common among businessmen who are constantly struggling to meet deadlines and push through deals. The third chakra is excessive and probably frustrated. The liver is swollen and excessive; the adrenals are overworked, exhausted, and contracted. The life force, housed in the kidneys, is tired, meaning both the kidneys and the second chakra are weak and deficient. For such a person, life is an ongoing struggle for survival among the fittest.

Occasionally you will see a person whose posture is fairly straight and relaxed except for a small paunch around and below the belt and a slightly concave solar plexus. Generally, there are two types of people with this posture: one person is considerably overweight and quite round; the other is tall, thin (except for the paunch in the stomach), and lank. In both types, the second chakra is weak and deficient, which suggests prostate problems (in men) and ovarian problems (in women). It also reveals swollen large intestines and weak elimination. The weak solar plexus area, coupled with the deficient second chakra, suggests a person with a very weak will, but that manifests quite differently in the two different statures, especially among men. The round man is usually jolly, positive, and satisfied with his lot. The tall, lank man is typically dissatisfied but highly repressed. He doesn't think much about his circumstances. It's as if something inside has been turned off. He's surrendered the struggle to grow or succeed. He's getting by; he doesn't enjoy much of anything fully, and he gives the impression of being asleep on some level.

*   *   *

In general, excesses of energy and deficiencies tend to balance each other and work as opposites. Very often, excesses of energy, blockages, and boulders appear in places of acute tension, such as the shoulders, the neck, the head, and the pelvis. Deficiencies are common in the chest, lungs, heart, and sex organs. Sometimes the right side of the body is excessive while the left is deficient, or vice versa. Often, you will find that the liver is excessive (on the right side of the body, just beneath the ribs) while the spleen/pancreas (on the left in the same area) is deficient.

Whenever you see imbalances in the posture, use your hands to explore the field closely. Concentrate and feel the energy with your entire being. Search the field with your hands, heart, and mind to determine where the blockages are and where the deficiencies and holes are located. Feel the tension in the field; feel the temperature changes, the boulders, and the holes. Trust your intuition and sense of touch, but be humble. Gently ask the person whether he or she suffers from digestive problems, if you see the possibility of intestinal imbalances, or heart palpitations, if you see deficiencies or excesses in the heart. When you sense an imbalance in the heart chakra, do not assume that the person has heart disease. Always ask the person if he or she suffers from any symptoms in the areas in which you sense problems, and if so, ask the person to see a physician.

When the Two Become One

During healing touch, you and the person with whom you are working share the same life energy. I have found that this sharing is very much a two-way street and that information passes back and forth between you during your session. This communication occurs in different ways. During the session, you may experience certain symptoms in your body, such as sudden movement, spasm, heat, tingling, prickly sensations, and mild pain. Very often, these symptoms appear in you because you are so attuned to the recipient's body and energetic field that you are reacting to the treatment as he or she is. Changes occurring in the recipient's field and body are reflected in yours, though on a much more reduced and very temporary scale. These experiences can guide you in your work. If you feel it is appropriate, tell the recipient of healing touch what you are feeling and ask if he or she is experiencing similar symptoms. At the same time, do not become attached to the pain or sensation, since it is generally not organic in your system. If you didn't have any similar sensations while you were centering, it is unlikely that they originated in your body. Thank these feelings for guiding you and release them as you exhale. As you become a more seasoned practitioner, you will no longer need to feel such symptoms in your body as a guide.

Another way in which information passes back and forth between you is through images or symbols that appear suddenly in your mind, as they did when I treated Wendy. The mind is not restricted to the brain, but also resides in the field. During healing touch, you are within this person's field; you are touching her mind. Powerful images that have shaped the recipient's life are still stored in her psyche and can pass easily from her field to yours and then suddenly become conscious to you. You might even experience the same thoughts and emotions as the recipient, including sudden feelings of fear, discomfort, or anger.

I cannot stress enough how important it is to center yourself at the outset of every treatment and to remain centered throughout the treatment. Whenever you experience images or emotions during a treatment, redouble your concentration by focusing on your prayer. This will protect you throughout the treatment and afterward.

I avoid discussing any image or emotion that I experience during the session with my client until I feel that we have established a bond of trust. The amount of time it takes to develop such a bond varies widely from person to person, of course, and only you can determine the right time for such a discussion. The essential point is that you should avoid jumping to conclusions after you have experienced this exchange of information. Such interpretations have to be correct, first of all, and shared at a time when the client is prepared to hear and accept such information. Wait for the right moment and then share the experience in a very gentle and unassuming way. The best way is simply to ask the person if the image you saw, or the feeling you experienced, has any resonance with him. You might ask the person: Do you relate at all to this image (or feeling)? If he says no, then file the experience in your memory. He may bring up the subject again when he is prepared to speak about it, or you may have a clearer insight into your experience later on that may be useful in your treatment.

We must remember the axiom I stated in chapter 1: Being a healer makes its greatest demands on the healer and not on the client. Your work as a practitioner of healing touch will force you to grow, and grow rapidly, in part because you will be confronting issues in others that will trigger the same or different issues in you. A person who has a terminal disease will cause you personal fears; the recipient who has undergone traumas that you find abhorrent will move you strongly; the client whom you dislike will make you face old wounds inside yourself. Everyone on whom you practice will present you with a challenge that is entirely your own, because each of those people will make you face yourself. Each person on whom you work becomes your teacher, and should be so revered.

Grounding the Patient by "Opening the Feet"

At the conclusion of the assessment process comes a step I call "opening the feet," or allowing the energy that is flowing down through the body to exit the feet and unify with the earth. This step provides a deep sense of physical, psychological, and spiritual stability to the person on whom you are working. It also allows energy that is backed up and blocked in the upper part of the body to be released. This step alone often harmonizes the entire field and can

relieve many painful symptoms in the upper body, especially headaches, because it draws the energy down from the upper part of the
body and field and into the lower parts.

Most people perform more mental labor than physical each
day. To support this work, their energy shifts from the lower parts
of the physical body to the upper, especially to the head, neck, and
shoulders. In addition, stress causes the sympathetic nervous system to shift energy and nerve innervation to the periphery of the
body to support the physical reactions associated with the well-
known flight-or-fight response. Thus, intellectual work and stress
combine to move the energy away from the center of being and into
the body's periphery, especially to the brain. This creates energetic
imbalances. The upper part of the body, such as the shoulders,
neck, and upper arms, can become excessive and stagnant, while
organs in the center of the body, such as the liver, stomach, digestive tract, and sex organs, can become deficient and weak. (For
more on the kinds of imbalances created by stress, see chapter 9.)
Therefore, I try to draw the energy from the upper and peripheral
parts of the body to the internal and lower parts by opening the
feet. This is how it is done:

Once I have reached the bottoms of the legs in my assessment,
I gently massage the muscles and tendons behind the knees, especially the points directly in the center behind the knees—the site of
secondary chakras, you will recall. I massage the site in a slow,
consistent fashion. This is the first and sometimes the only time I
touch the physical body. After a few minutes of gently massaging
the back of the knee, I gradually move down the calf and on to the
Achilles tendon and then to the bottom of the foot of the same leg,
massaging deeply, gently, and rhythmically. (I work on each leg
and foot individually.)

While I do this work, I consciously try to pull the energy down
from the upper part of the body into the lower legs and feet. You
will recall from chapter 3 how we practiced pulling the energy from
one part of the body and pushing it to another. Here, I visualize
pulling the energy from the head, chest, abdomen, hips, and thighs,

and sending it down into the calf muscle, Achilles tendon, and bottom of the foot. This massage and pulling of energy centers the person, balances the energy throughout the body, and stabilizes the patient's field.

I then attempt to "open the feet" by holding the secondary chakras at the arches of the feet. This will allow the energy that I have brought down into the feet to flow out and make its natural link with the earth, thus giving the person a sense of being "grounded," or physically and psychologically stable.

I do this by placing my middle finger on the arch of the foot and massaging gently. At first, I try to sense the subtle energy emerging from the foot. I try to determine if the energy is flowing out of the secondary chakra on the bottom of the foot, as it should, or if it is blocked. You can often feel the stagnation of the energy within the foot because the skin itself feels tight, thick, or hard. Sometimes the bottoms of the feet feel inert, almost wooden, rather than supple and alive. If the energy is blocked, I ask the client to breathe deeply and try to visualize the life force moving into the body with each breath and then down into the feet. On the out breath, the person should visualize the energy moving out of the bottoms of the feet and into the earth. Meanwhile, I hold my hand on the foot, at the arch, and feel myself pulling the energy down into the feet as the patient inhales. I also visualize the secondary chakras at the arch opening and becoming active and revitalized. As the patient exhales, I visualize the energy moving out of the feet and rejoining the earth. I do the same with both feet.

No matter what I sense when I touch the feet, I always try to open the chakras at the feet by gently massaging the arches and pulling the energy down and out of the foot. I then hold the foot at the arch until the energy changes, which can take five to ten minutes.

All of this work has a significant effect on the recipient because, in effect, I have literally directed his consciousness and life force to the areas where I wanted it. Remember, I did not touch the person's physical body until I began massaging the backs of the patient's knees. I then began to work on the calves, tendons, and feet. This pattern of touching the knees, calves, and feet directs the person's awareness first to the backs of the knees and then down to the calves, tendons, and into the feet. By doing that, I am directing his life energy in the same way—downward and ultimately to the secondary chakras at the arches. I am not merely visualizing the movement of energy, but literally directing the patient to move his own energy to the places within the body where I want it. By asking the patient to "breathe into the feet" and visualize the energy moving with the breath, I am also utilizing the person's natural ability to move his own energy. Thus, we are working together to move his consciousness and the life force back into the body and reunite it with the earth.

After I have held one foot for a time and "feel" with my entire being the flow of energy leaving the foot, I perform the same exercise on the other foot, and once again ask the recipient to visualize the energy penetrating deeply into the feet from the rest of the body on the inhalation and out of the feet on the exhalation.

When I am sure that the energy is flowing through the feet, I resume the first position, with my hands over the recipient's head. I then slowly but steadily run my hands over the recipient's field once again to determine how the energy has changed. Each time a healing touch practitioner passes his or her hands through a recipient's field, he or she has changed that energy field.

In the meanwhile, I have forgotten myself entirely in the process. I am thinking of nothing but my prayer, but the prayer allows me to be empty. It gives my mind something to do, something to be occupied with, while my higher self directs my actions. Now I am ready to work on the field.

Associative Ideas

The practice of any traditional healing therapy inevitably leads you into an exploration of other ancient practices, which, you will find, share many underlying themes. Healing touch is consistent with and even shares many of the same principles of other ancient therapies, especially Chinese medicine. The more I study Chinese medicine, the more impressed I am with its insight into the nature of health and disease, the efficacy of its methods of treatment, and its ability to understand the relationship between the body and the mind. It is this latter understanding that can be so helpful to you, particularly when assessing the origin of particular health problems. Nothing within Chinese medicine better articulates the relationship between body and mind better than the Theory of the Five Elements.

More than two thousand years ago, ancient Chinese sages developed a system that has come to be known as the Theory of the Five Elements, which is a complex but powerful healing tool. Among the important aspects of the theory is the association of specific emotions and psychological states within certain parts of the body. The Chinese found that particular types of emotions were grounded in certain individual organs. As the Chinese saw it, the mind was grounded in the body and depended on the health of the body for the proper functioning of the psyche. As long as the organ is healthy, the Chinese sages said, these emotions and psychological states will remain in balance. Hence, the equilibrium of the mind depends upon the health of the body.

After more than fifteen years of practice, I have found that the Chinese were right in their association of organs and emotions. The more imbalanced the liver is, for example, the more a person is prone to anger. The more imbalanced the heart, the less joy and laughter a person experiences. My experience has also given me additional insights into the link between organs and emotional states. Below is a list of organs and their associated psychological conditions; it is based on the Chinese system, my own experience, and research. Use this list as a loose guide in your own practice and, specifically, in your assessment of your client's field. Discover for yourself if these associations are true. I have deliberately kept them short to serve as springboards to your own intuition and creativity. The idea is not to get locked into these associations but to use them as a guide for exploration and study. Also, notice how your recipient's emotional condition changes as his or her health improves.

The list provides the characteristics people experience when the organ is generally balanced and healthy, as well as the characteristics that dominate the personality when the organ is imbalanced and suffers from some disorder. It's important to note that all of us, from time to time, experience the characteristics that are associated with imbalance. What you should be looking for when you do your assessment of a client are the characteristics that dominate the personality and profoundly shape the person's outlook on life.

ORGAN	PERSONALITY CHARACTERISTICS WHEN ORGAN IS BALANCED	EMOTIONS AND PSYCHOLOGY WHEN SIGNIFICANTLY IMBALANCED
LIVER	Strong ability to express strong will; good	Anger, frustration, weak will, inability to express oneself, overly timid
SPLEEN	Good self-esteem, centered personality, lack of worry, compassion and understanding	Worry, anxiety, nervousness
STOMACH	Strong appetite for life, good ability to enjoy a wide variety of people and types of experience	Nervous; poor appetite for life; very picky about food, people, and types of experiences he or she can tolerate

HEART	Can give and feel love, can identify with others, can feel connected to others	Walls self off from love and affection, feels isolated and tends to sustain isolation, may be given to hysteria, depression, low self-esteem
PANCREAS	Good sense of boundaries	Suffers from chronic guilt
GALL-BLADDER	Decisive, good digestion	Indecisive, poor digestion
SMALL INTESTINE	Can determine what is good in experience and what should be discarded	Has trouble finding the good in people, situations, and one's own experience in life
SKIN	Good sense of boundaries, positive sense of self, good self-esteem, good elimination from kidneys and large intestine	Weak sense of boundaries; poor self-esteem and sense of self; poor elimination from kidneys, bladder, and large intestine
LARGE INTESTINE	Able to let go of the past, not overly burdened by sadness or grief	Constipation: holding on to old memories, sadness, and grief; unable to let go of old hurts; trouble letting go of the past Diarrhea: unable to get the most out of experience. Lets go too easily of people and relationships

THYROID	Good self-expression	Hypothyroid: low energy and generally weak self-expression
		Hyperthyroid: racing, unable to deeply appreciate the moment or one's own contributions to an endeavor
SEX ORGANS	Good expression of one's own unique self and creativity	Holding back one's expression and creativity
KIDNEYS	Confident and generally secure personality	Suffers from deep-rooted fears
LUNGS	Good energy and vitality, strong ability to take in and enjoy life	Repressed emotions, low energy (oxygen is the basis for energy), low self-esteem, strong sense of one's own weakness or frailty

Everything Is Searching for Balance

The body, mind, and spirit are always searching for balance in all ways, especially energetically. Whenever you see excessive strength, you will also discover weakness nearby. Always look for the paired opposites. Once you discover the imbalance, you will want to move the energy from the area of excess to the places where it is deficient.

A practitioner of healing touch is always trying to restore balance to the body, mind, and spirit.

If you keep these guidelines in your mind as you are doing your assessment, you will be able to know where the blockages in the field lie, even if you cannot "feel" the energy as yet.

EXERCISE—THREE POINT MEDITATION

As you recall, we have mentioned that it is the whole field that becomes charged with energy from the universal source before the energy work. The healer works as a whole unit. The hands can merely direct and be specific with the energy.

The first part of the following exercise teaches you to use your own field to reach out and "scan" the other person, and the second part teaches you to send healing energy through your field to the other person.

This exercise can be done with two or more people. If there are more than two people, pick the person who is going to be scanned and have him or her sit in the middle with the rest of the group forming a circle around him or her. (See diagram 3-Point Meditation in the color insert.)

1. Start this exercise by using the meditative clearing exercise from chapter 1, choosing one person to guide the imagery. Picture the sun or source over the center of the whole group, not over each one individually. Do this for about five minutes.

    The person who has been chosen to guide this meditation will now guide the rest through the imagery.

    •   The person in the center should focus on what he needs to heal within any part of his body, emotion, or mind, while also keeping himself centered in his egg or bubble (see the egg meditation, page 140).

    •   The rest of the group should be centered in their individual energy eggs and begin to move their energy from the front of their eggs to gently make contact with the person in the center of the circle in a neutral energy mode. Stay here for five minutes and just feel or get a sense of what is going on with this person. Note any images you have, any physical sensations, any thoughts, etc.

After five minutes, gently withdraw your energy. Open your eyes and have each person in the group share with the person in the center what each received. The person in the center should also share what he received. Remember that you have been in the center person's sacred space. Not only is this information confidential within the group, but you have been privy to secrets within the person and you should be gentle with how you share the thoughts. Remember that the purpose of healing touch is "to help and to heal" from a nonjudgmental place.

Chat for a short time. Some associations may have *no* relevance at the time. That happens.

2. In the same circle, center yourselves again by breathing. The person in the center should open himself to receive healing energies. The group should bring healing energy from the source through each to the center person through each individual field. Continue this for about five minutes. Your energy is in the "gentle push" stage. At the end of five minutes, consciously feel your energy go into neutral and withdraw your energy from the center person's sacred space.

Each one takes a turn being in the middle, each being supportive of the other.

It is important to remember that when you are in another's sacred space, you know everything about that person. It may not be conscious in you, but on some level there is a great awareness. You must remember not only to be nonjudgmental but to honor this space as you would your own.

8

Working on the Field

Barbara came to me in July 1988 suffering from terrible migraine headaches that kept her in bed about once a week, on average. Sometimes the symptoms that accompanied the headaches—nausea, vomiting, sensitivity to light, and aching shoulders and back—would force her to remain in bed for four or five days. She also endured chronic low back pain, fibroid tumors, ovarian pain (especially at the time of her periods), premenstrual syndrome (PMS), and the early stages of an ulcer that gave her periodic stomach pains. She was in her early thirties, recently married, with no children. One of the things I noticed immediately was Barbara's lack of confidence. She was nervous and distinctly uncomfortable talking about herself. Clearly, she needed help, especially for her migraines, but she seemed reluctant to share her pain with me or, as I would eventually learn, with anyone.

It didn't take me long to realize that Barbara's lack of confidence was central to her physical problems. She grew up as the oldest of five children, her siblings all boys. Her mother relied heavily on Barbara to help raise her brothers. By the time she was ten, she was changing diapers and baby-sitting. Responsibility came early in life for Barbara, and the pattern of focusing on the needs of others rather than her own eventually became a character trait that marked her adult life.

"I didn't think of this as a problem," Barbara recalled many years later. "When I was young, I learned to cook because I wanted to. I wanted to take care of my brothers. I always thought of them as the 'little guys.' I never thought that someone should be taking care of me or that I should be taking care of me. I didn't realize how much this way of thinking was driving me and causing my life to be so imbalanced."

Such a mentality, which is so common today, gives rise to a lifestyle that requires an enormous amount of energy. Barbara was constantly trying to meet the needs of others. Her sense of self-worth and even of her own safety was predicated on removing the discomforts of her husband, her friends, and those with whom she worked. Unconsciously, Barbara felt responsible for making right every situation in which she found herself.

Barbara is a classic example of how holes in the field shape a person's life, and how one compensates for the energy leaks. Her field was so riddled with holes that she had no clear sense of boundaries or identity, and thus she could not discern the needs of others versus her own needs. This identification with others, in fact, is dangerous to one's health, because the person with such a problem is unable to establish any sort of balance in his or her life.

"I was trying to be superwoman," Barbara recalls. "I had to please everyone. I had no sense of my own boundaries or my own limits. I was constantly engulfed by my surroundings. I couldn't block them out."

On the day that Barbara showed up at my office, she was suffering from a dull headache that she was afraid might become a migraine. She also had low backache. After conducting the initial interview with Barbara, I recommended dietary changes—especially a significant reduction in fat and sugar to help reduce the premenstrual symptoms (diets high in fat are associated with more intense PMS due largely to the secretion of estrogen from fat cells; high estrogen levels increase the symptoms of PMS). I also recommended a series of supplements that would support her liver and digestive functions.

Then I began a series of healing touch sessions because I wanted to help her relax and experience her own center. Despite her problems, Barbara responded quickly.

I began the work by doing an assessment. As I passed my hands through her field, I sensed tension, tightness, and a kind of spiky, tingling sensation. "Are you tense?" I asked her. "I'm feeling pretty mad right now," Barbara said. "I just had a run-in with my boss and I can't think straight. I can't talk about it."

Whenever a person is angry and tense, the diaphragm (or third chakra) tends to tighten and cause the breathing to become shallow. Thus, I knew that the first chakra (self-protection and survival issues), second (sex organs), third, and sixth (headaches) were troubled and needed work.

With Barbara, I began by opening the secondary chakras in her feet to drain the backed-up energy in the entire system. After I had gently massaged her arches, I held both of her feet for about five minutes, meanwhile asking her to breathe deeply, slowly, and rhythmically into her feet. Next, I sent healing energy to her second and third chakras. I then worked on the periphery of her field, closing over the holes, thus giving her a greater sense of her own boundary.

Usually opening the feet drains the energy that has been stuck in the upper part of the body and reduces or eliminates headaches. This worked for Barbara, but I noticed during my assessment toward the end of the session that her sixth chakra still felt dull and deficient of life force. To support the energy in the sixth chakra, I placed my left hand over the field at the back of her head (not touching the skin) and my right hand over her forehead area, and then visualized healing energy clearing Barbara's head. I did not send energy through my hands. Headaches are an indication of blocked energy within the body, including the head. You do not want to add to the congestion by sending more energy to the area. Rather, I used my hands to pull stagnation out of the chakra, head, and neck region. Meanwhile, I also envisioned the energy circulating more freely in the chakra, head, and upper body. Usually, this was enough to relieve Barbara's headaches, but if it didn't, I would often return to Barbara's feet and open the secondary chakras again, holding the arches for about five minutes.

"I was amazed at how good I felt after that first session with Deby," Barbara recalled. "I felt as if someone had lifted twenty pounds of weight off my back. I had a great sense of relief."

I did energy work on Barbara regularly, usually once a week or twice a month. Gradually, her symptoms began to diminish, until eventually they disappeared.

"As I started to receive healing touch regularly, I began to realize that this was working. At first, it was some internal knowing, more intuitive than anything, but pretty soon my health was improving. The first sign was that my migraines were not as intense as before. And then I no longer got them as frequently. I went from having a migraine once a week to twice a month. Then I'd go a whole month without a migraine, and that was something."

Besides the diminished migraine symptoms, Barbara had no ovarian pain. Remarkably, after four months of healing touch, doctors could no longer find Barbara's ovarian cysts. Gone, too, were her intense PMS and her digestive distress. It took us more than a year to get the migraines completely under control, but Barbara has not experienced a migraine in two years. Occasionally, she'll experience a tension headache that is quickly relieved by over-the-counter medication. Meanwhile, she's learning how to let go of her tension on her own, as she is becoming increasingly aware of her own energetic patterns.

"Healing touch has helped me to sit down, calm myself, and relax enough to let the tension release," says Barbara. "It lets me experience being in a peaceful internal space, a place where I can leave my family and work outside the door and focus on my own needs. The work is meditative and it's very supportive. The process has really been about getting to know myself. Part of that means knowing how I'm feeling. Now, if I have a headache coming on, I recognize the tension well in advance and I start breathing and allowing my body to relax. I'm learning to let go of my tension."

Improvement in Barbara's physical health has not been the only blessing of healing touch, however. She has undergone a remarkable transformation in her demeanor, attitudes, and self-understanding. As Barbara and I regularly began to work together, she started to see the connection between her low self-esteem and her need to please others. "I was just trying to be loved," she says today. As her energetic field got stronger and her sense of self improved, she naturally began to appreciate herself more and more. "I began to get a glimpse of the person I could be, and that started to feel really good," Barbara said. Much of this, Barbara maintains, has come about because she has learned to turn her focus inward, to the self within.

"Since I began this practice, I have gradually evolved beyond the old mind-set," said Barbara.

In Service to Others, Less Is Often More

After assessing a person's physical and energetic bodies, I start to work on the field, usually at a distance of about eighteen inches, a distance that is traditionally known as the sacred space. Within this area, a person's sensitivity and self-protectiveness are more acute, and consequently you do not want to violate this space, especially during the first few treatments, because you may not yet have established a bond of trust. Even when I work on people I am very familiar with, I still try to remain beyond the eighteen-inch boundary during our first two sessions together. The obvious contradiction to this is my touching of the secondary chakras at the backs of the knees and my massaging the backs of the legs, the tendons in the calves, and the bottoms of the feet. This work, which I call opening the feet, is so important to balancing a person's energy that there simply is no way around it. Nevertheless, I approach the body and these secondary chakras with great respect and appreciation for this person and his willingness to allow me to work with him.

Opening the feet is performed at the conclusion of the assessment. Once that is done, I start at the top of the field and move downward toward the feet. I am aware of the energy flowing to me from the cosmos, above, and the earth, below. I feel the energy passing from my field, to my body, up from my heart, and down to my hands. My hands are flowing with healing energy as I pass them over the patient's field.

The first and most important part of the work is to be an instrument for universal life force. That energy is flowing through me and into the person I am working with. It's that simple. Thus, the very basis of the practice requires very little from me, because the life force flowing from the Universal Healer is doing the healing. I am attempting to direct and facilitate that flow of energy from an infinite source to the person in need of assistance. As I tell my students, once a practitioner recognizes and achieves this standpoint, she is in a position to help a person. Her ego is out of the way and cannot be an obstruction to the process. This is what I mean when I say "less is more."

As I send life force to the field, I am particularly conscious of the places in the field that I had perceived to be imbalanced while doing my assessment, or where a symptom may be manifesting. Of course, I do not have to perceive blockages or holes in the field to recognize and treat a broken arm or a physical wound or some form of disorder. I can treat the imbalance by sending life energy to that part of the body. That is the beauty of healing touch: At bottom, I am sending loving, healing energy. The body and the Great Spirit together know better than I what to do with that energy.

Unblocking the Rivers: Removing Stones and Boulders

In general, all symptoms arise out of imbalance. Either there is too much energy in the area or too little. As a general rule, you are trying to move the excess energy into the places where there is deficiency, as I did in chapter 2, where I reported on my work with Wendy.

Once I discover an imbalance in the energy field, I focus on it and attempt to restore circulation of the life force to that area. If the area is blocked, or stagnant, I try to gently remove the obstruction—often perceived as a large stone, or boulder—from that part of the field. These boulders are perceived as large, dense clumps of energy.

I have found that before you try to remove blockages from the field, it's helpful to ask the person with whom you are working to visualize the energy within her body flowing freely, without obstruction, especially the energy that flows up and down the central tube.

Visualization: Encouraging the Free Flow of Energy Within the Patient

Ask your patient to visualize the following as you are doing your energy work: Picture yourself under a waterfall of the richest, most powerful, life-restoring energy. You can feel the energy wash over and through you, entering your pores, fibers, and cells. Notice that each droplet of energy sparkles light; each droplet is packed with photons of energy; they radiate with all the colors of the rainbow. Notice that your every cell drinks up these droplets of Qi like a thirsty traveler who's been too long in the desert. Breathe in the energy and draw it into every cell and every dark or weakened crevice of your body. Inhale the energy deeply so that it enters the top of your head. All the energy that you need is absorbed fully so that you have an abundance of life force within you. You are fully nourished from an infinite source. All you need is available to you at any moment. As you exhale, visualize all that you don't need being released through the soles of your feet and into the earth to be transformed by the Great Mother.

As the person performs this visualization, begin to remove the blockages in the field.

*   *   *

Whenever you perceive a blockage in the field, visualize it as a big stone in the river of energy that supplies that part of the body with life force. See the eddies, whirlpools, and vortices that manifest in the field around and directly over the injury or disorder in the physical body. Remember that excesses of energy and deficiencies tend to appear in tandem, so that an excess in one part of the body will create a deficiency somewhere else. Excesses of energy, blockages, and boulders appear in places of acute tension, such as the shoulders, the neck, the head, and the pelvis. Deficiencies are common in the chest, lungs, heart, and sex organs.

I try to free the area of a boulder, or chaotic energy (sometimes perceived as static electricity), or stagnant energy (often perceived as dense resistance) by "grasping" and "removing" it with my hands. As I reach into the area of the boulder, I move my hand in a counterclockwise direction and cup my hand to grasp the obstruction. I move my hand out of the field in a clockwise motion. I then release that energy upward into the Light of Love, to be transmuted by the Universal Healer. In places where the energy is turbulent and chaotic, I "smooth" the field, and try to calm it, by giving it healing, even maternal, care. I do this by stroking the field in a calming and loving manner. Wherever I perceive stagnant energy, which is usually excessive energy, I try to move it to a place where the energy is deficient by using the technique of "pulling" the energy, as I described in chapter 3.

To remove blockages from a chakra area, reach into the field at the site of the blockage while moving your hand in a counterclockwise direction. As you move counterclockwise, you are moving healing energy into the area. See your hand grasping the bolus of energy, or stone, from the whirlpool and lifting it from the field. As you retract your hand and pull the stone from the field, turn your hand in a clockwise direction. The clockwise direction facilitates the movement of aberrant energy out of the body.

Once your hand and the stone are free, lift them up to the ceiling and say to yourself: "I release this which she/he no longer needs into the Light of Love." Feel the energy go off your palm and upward, to be transformed. Then say: "I return my hand bringing peace and harmony to my vibral core." You do this so that none of the aberrant energy returns to you. (It is inherent in your treatment and your prayer that you are bringing peace and harmony to the recipient.)

Do the same if you are working with someone whom you perceive to carry a great deal of anger, rage, or intense emotion in the field. When you remove obstructions in the field—which may be accumulations of stagnant emotions—you should release them into the Light of Love. Once that is done, shake off any residual energy from your hands and release that into the Light of Love as well. This will protect you. You will find that even after you have worked on several clients in the same day, you will still feel light and unaffected by their emotional states.

While you are removing disharmonies from the field with your right hand, hold your left on the other side of the patient to maintain balance. Your left hand acts as a stabilizer to his field, while your right removes old or stagnant forms of energy.

Reassess the field and note any changes that have occurred. Repeat the process until all vestiges of stagnation and tension have been eliminated.

If you perceive that the energy is still deficient in the area in which you have worked, move your hand to the nearest chakra and place one hand in front of the chakra and the other behind the patient's back in the general area where the same chakra exits at the spine. Your hands are now opposite each other and the patient is between them. Now build an energy ball between your hands and feel that part of the body expand and become balanced with life energy.

Closing Holes

A vitally important task for the practitioner of healing touch is to close holes, or leaks, in the field. This will allow the person to experience, even for a short time, his or her true wholeness and integrity, an experience that triggers the healing process. Once the patient glimpses his best self, he unconsciously and consciously begins to move out of stasis and stagnation. The more you work on a person, the more you can "repattern" the field to close the leaks permanently, or teach the person to close the leaks whenever he feels vulnerable.

Typically, holes or leaks occur near areas of the field that are loaded with energy, often stuck or blocked from flowing into the hole. The field will try to heal itself of leaks, but blockages may prevent the life force from flowing smoothly to the hole or leak. Leaks are often near those chakras that are related to the kinds of issues the person may be experiencing. (Those issues may well have been discussed during your intake interview or as part of the healing session.) If it's an issue around money, for example, then perhaps the hole is located near the first chakra—responsible for survival issues, or the third chakra—responsible for the will and drive, or the fifth chakra—responsible for self-expression. If the issue involves relationships with the opposite sex, then perhaps it involves the second chakra—responsible for sexuality, or the third chakra—responsible for will and self-empowerment, or the fourth chakra—responsible for the ability to experience love. If the issue involves the discovery of the person's specific work, then perhaps it involves the second chakra—responsible for creativity, or the fourth chakra—responsible for discerning what it is the person truly loves, or the fifth chakra—responsible for self-expression, or the sixth chakra—responsible for one's deep understanding of self.

If the person has come to you complaining of a specific health issue, search the field around the nearest related chakra. If you do not feel a leak or a hole, reassess the field and open the feet. You may need to spend five minutes of the treatment holding the feet and encouraging the person to breathe deeply down into the feet. (Very often, people who are difficult to assess are shallow breathers and, consequently, suffer from stagnant life energy. These imbalances can very often be relieved by asking the person to spend five minutes breathing deeply while you are opening the secondary chakras in their feet.) Be patient with your assessment. It may take several sessions before you understand the person's energetic imbalances. Meanwhile, you are harmonizing the field through your healing touch and by opening the chakras in the feet.

To close off the holes and leaks, I run my hands along boundaries of the field that are healthy and strong and draw the excess energy to the hole or leak. I try to channel additional life force to the hole, filling it with energy, and then close over the wounded area by smoothing my hands over the leak. I give the leak a kind of maternal love; flowing within that love is the healing energy that is flowing through me to the client. I visualize the healing energy flowing into the leak, filling it, and healing the wound. I "see" the wound closing and the integrity of the field being reestablished. I work to balance the energy so that it flows smoothly throughout the region where there was formerly a wound. Once again, the field is closed, strong, resilient, and whole.

The process of closing a leak or hole usually takes several sessions, simply because wounds are usually chronic and the field is patterned to maintain that wound.

When holes or leaks in the field are closed, even if only temporarily, the person experiences a feeling of wholeness. His field is now intact, and energy that was leaking is now flowing within him. This experience may give him a sudden burst of energy or it may make him feel tired, as areas of his body are experiencing energy for the first time in many years. But more important, body, mind, and spirit feel *contained* within one's own boundaries and identity. The effect is profound, because it reminds one on all levels of what it feels like to be whole; it is a glimpse of all that one is and can be. That experience catalyzes the entire being and all the healing forces that exist within. Energies are shaken out of their stasis and awakened to the fact that the field has been wounded and must be healed. In effect, the psyche has been roused and mobilized in a specific direction. The full self-healing of those holes takes place long after the session is over. The person's own field will heal itself. The closing of the holes by the practitioner awakens the healing forces within the field and directs them to those places within the field that must be restored to integrity.

When Someone Complains of Pain

Occasionally, someone will tell you that she or he is experiencing a mild ache or pain after a treatment. If the pain is acute and/or lingers for more than two hours, ask the person to see a physician. In general, you cannot cause any serious side effect—including pain—by administering healing touch. On the other hand, the infusion of the life force can create temporary discomfort, especially in the person who has suffered long-term blockages and stagnation.

The most common pain that may result after a healing touch session occurs after you have cleared an area of obstructions and old energetic patterns begin to break down. Once these blockages are removed, energy, blood, and lymph flow in greater abundance into areas that were previously blocked and deficient of all three elixirs of life. When blood, lymph, and Qi start to move into parts of the field and physical body that were stagnant or blocked, the tissues can be highly sensitive and therefore might experience temporary discomfort or mild pain.

Whenever a client experiences pain—but especially if that pain emerges after a treatment—first open the feet. If there is still pain after opening the feet, place your hands over the site of the pain and send that place soothing, comforting, and healing energy. Visualize the tissues opening, as if they were just now arising after a long sleep, and accepting the increased circulation. Once you have done this, move one hand over the nearest chakra's opening and place the other hand over the back where the chakra exits. Now, create a new energy ball between your hands. See the energy ball fill up the entire area with soft, healing energy and light. See the tissues becoming supple and relaxed. Finally, make sure the energy is flowing freely from the bottoms of the feet.

Balancing the Chakras

After the treatment has been completed, ask the patient to lie down on a table or on a mat on the floor and reassess the field, especially concentrating on what you are feeling when your hands go over the seven chakra areas. Try to balance any disharmonies that may remain. If one or more of the chakras is still weak, you can build the chakra's life force by doing the following. Move to the right side of the client's body. Place your left hand under the client's back, at the exit point of the chakra in question, and your right hand over the front of the same imbalanced chakra. For this treatment, you will have to touch the person on his or her back and/or front at the site of the chakra on which you are working. Visualize the Universal Energy moving through you. See the energy entering your field and your body through the top of your head. Draw in the life force with your breath. As you exhale, see the energy flow up from your heart into your shoulders, arms, and hands. Finally, see the life force building between your hands. You are creating an energy ball, a sphere of life force, between your hands in the chakra that needs healing. As you are filling the chakra with this powerful ball of light, repeat the phrase "To help and to heal" over and over again in your mind. (See Appendix 2 photos.)

One of the signs that the chakra is accepting the energy and being healed is that you will hear gurgling sounds emanating from the stomach and bowels (similar to the growling sounds of a hungry stomach). This indicates that the additional energy being channeled into the field is clearing the stagnation within the chakra and other places in the field and that new additional life force is moving into the body, clearing it of stagnation, and restoring harmony.

Hold the chakra ball for as long as you think is necessary. Intuitively, you will know how long to hold the ball of energy. You will feel the moment when you know the sphere of life force has been accepted into the person's field and body. It usually takes only a few minutes for the body and field to accept the chakra ball.

The purpose of balancing the chakras after the session is completed is to help the energy system accommodate the changes in patterning that have just occurred.

Once you have balanced the chakras, pass your hands through the field and visualize your hands smoothing, straightening, and closing the edges of the energy field. Close any holes or leaks in the field that you may still feel. Finally, groom the field, so to speak. Hold your left palm up at about shoulder height and with your right hand stroke the edges of the field as though you were smoothing all the fibers around that energetic ball of "cotton candy." Move vertically downward in a clockwise direction around the field with each stroke. It usually takes about seven strokes.

When this step is completed, ask the client to lie down for ten minutes. The energy that has been channeled to the client will build on itself over the next twenty-four hours, boosting the immune and healing forces and harmonizing imbalances. Ask the person to assist this process by maintaining a relaxed pace through the next day.

Expanded Integrated Awareness Begins with Remembering

Throughout this book, I have been reporting how people, when they begin healing touch, reintegrate repressed or forgotten parts of their being. I call this "expanded integrated awareness." That experience very often occurs because we hold memories, talents, and awareness in parts of the field that are blocked from our conscious minds. When a practitioner of healing touch begins to work on the disorder, he or she invariably removes many of these repressive barriers, thus freeing these memories and abilities, which are experienced by the person as a gradual awareness of self in a whole new light.

Before that awareness occurs, however, the person with whom you are working may remember and psychologically reexperience an old trauma. In order for the body, mind, and spirit to heal, the person very often revisits the memory of the events that caused the original wound. In fact, this is an essential part of the healing. That experience must be reintegrated into the psyche, especially if it has been repressed and denied for some time. Healing touch greatly assists the person to go back to those painful memories and makes the process of reintegration so much easier because the practitioner of healing touch is sending the client love in the form of healing energy to the very place where the client has been wounded. This place has been deprived of optimal amounts of life force, blood, and lymph for some time. These are the fundamental elements of life. Once these basics are restored, the client feels strong enough to go back to the pain and deal with it in a whole new way. Thus, the person returns to the scene of the crime, so to speak, this time holding the hand of divine love, which is being channeled to the patient from the practitioner.

Here is yet another area where healing touch can greatly assist the work of other health care providers, especially a mental health professional. If a person comes to you with a long-lasting emotional disorder, refer him or her to a psychologist or psychiatrist. Meanwhile, as you work on the field, be sure to keep the treatments short—usually no more than ten to fifteen minutes at each session. You can perform the treatments daily, however. At the same time, strongly urge the person to keep a diary or a journal, especially to write about the painful events in his or her life. Studies have shown that writing about one's life, and particularly about past traumas, has a dramatic healing effect on body, mind, and spirit.

At Southern Methodist University (SMU), James W. Pennebaker, Ph.D., a professor of psychology, has found that writing about traumatic experiences in one's personal journal for twenty minutes a day, for four consecutive days, has a remarkable healing effect both physically and psychologically. Pennebaker and fellow researchers Janice Kecolt-Glaser and Ronald Glaser have discovered that immune response and psychological health are greatly enhanced after confessing traumas to one's journal.

When the scientists compared the immune systems of people

who wrote about their problems to the immune systems of those who didn't, the writers were found to have far more aggressive CD4 cells, the cells that coordinate the immune system's overall response to a disease. In fact, those people whom Pennebaker termed "high disclosers" had the most remarkable improvement in T-cell response of all participants.

Moreover, writing was also shown to dramatically improve psychological health as measured by interviews and psychological testing.

Pennebaker maintains that more than mere catharsis is at work here. He suggests that psychological inhibition—the mechanism by which we keep things secret, even from ourselves—requires a certain degree of psychic and physical energy. As he puts it, inhibition is a demanding form of work, especially when a very painful trauma must be kept secret. Physical symptoms—such as elevations in blood pressure, heart rate, breathing, skin temperature, and perspiration levels—frequently occur as a result of such inhibition. The release that accompanies confession, therefore, occurs on both psychological and physical levels.

Pennebaker points out that one does not necessarily have to write down the event to experience release. Confessing it to someone else will have the same effect, as long as it was a distinct traumatic event that one has kept secret, in whole or in part, to that point.

The rules for writing such confessions are simple enough:

1. Write for twenty minutes, for four consecutive days.
2. Write continuously about the most upsetting experience or trauma of your entire life.
3. Don't worry about grammar, spelling, or the structure of the piece.
4. Write your deepest thoughts and emotions regarding the experience. Write all the details you remember. Write down your insights into the events. In the process, get in touch with your deepest emotions and thoughts.

In any case, revisiting the pain of a trauma is often an essential part of the healing process, and it can be very rewarding for the patient.

One of the most powerful tools for helping a person eliminate unhealthy habits and for reducing psychological pain is clearing the spiritual channel, or the central tube, which is what we'll discuss next.

9

Clearing Old Patterns

Our lives are made up of a series of experiences that, taken together, can be seen to form patterns that make each of us unique. We all are shaped by patterns of thought, outlooks on life, and our preferences for certain kinds of experiences. A multitude of attitudes and beliefs within each of us combines to form patterns that determine the kinds of people we like, those we love, and those we dislike and of whom we are afraid. Our talents, ambitions, and weaknesses coalesce into patterns that give direction to our lives. Patterns reveal where we are strong and what within us needs to mature and develop. Our appearance is a pattern of physical features. When examined honestly and with insight, our patterns can reveal to us who we are and how we fit in the world.

Some of the forces that shape us are genetic and are therefore either fixed or of limited flexibility. Many of our talents and abilities are genetically determined, for example. Others are created by our experiences and environment. How you relate to authority figures or the opposite sex, your attitudes about money, and your thoughts about yourself and God are patterns that arose, in part, from your conditioning, but they are also ever-changing. They may seem rigid, even to the point of being fixed, yet they are quite mutable and, potentially, subject to enormous transformation.

As everyone who's ever tried to change a negative pattern knows, the work isn't easy, and sometimes it can be downright excruciating. Why is change so difficult? we may ask. Why is it that we can see behavioral problems so clearly at times, and yet succumb to them over and over again? The fact is that change may begin in the mind—it may start with recognition—but the mind alone cannot create change. We all know this to be true because most of the changes that have taken place in our lives have been accomplished without conscious effort and even without recognition. It is true that maturation is painful at times, but it is rarely, if ever, a singularly mental function. If it was, none of us would emerge from puberty, or awaken from adolescence, simply because the mind is not equipped to navigate its way through such troubled waters. Yet, somehow most of us grow beyond these stages. We pass into adulthood and continue to evolve—sometimes consciously, most of the time unconsciously.

What, then, is the driving force behind change, and how does change occur? In Ecclesiastes, the Preacher tells us: "There is an appointed time for everything. And there is a time for every event under heaven . . ." This suggests not only that "to everything . . . there is a season," as the Byrds' 1960s song "Turn! Turn! Turn!" so nicely put it, but that each event has its own purpose according to some larger plan. Change comes at its appointed time, says the Preacher, and is ordained by God. Why, then, is change so difficult?

When we examine nature, we find that change is occurring all the time. Many of the most profound changes are both smooth and orderly—so orderly, in fact, that we even set our calendars by them. In temperate climates, for example, nature makes four dramatic transformations annually, each according to its time. Insofar as we know, the tree does not think that it is now autumn and therefore time to let go of its leaves; or summer and therefore time to let out its fruit. Something else takes place that permits the tree to undergo such a remarkable transformation. That something is a change in the energy of the tree. In the fall, the life force of a tree turns downward and brings with it the sap, causing the leaves to fall off their limbs for lack of energy to support their lives. In winter, the energy stays below ground; it waits for the moment when the rising energy of spring will cause the life force of the tree to rise. Then the sun returns and the life energy rises through the trunk and flows into the branches and sprouts blossoms and leaves. In summer, the periphery of the tree is bursting with energy; all of nature is exploding with the life force, and so there are flowers and fruit.

Humans change in similar ways, and each of the changes we experience has its own season. Still, we have the power to alter the energy flowing through us with our thoughts, emotions, food, and behavior. We can promote the life force, or we can cause it to be blocked and stagnate. Most of the time, we do this without realizing it. Yet, no change takes place inside of us—no matter how hard we try—until there has been a dramatic energetic shift within. Once the energy in the field has changed—just as the energy within a tree has changed—our lives make some dramatic shift on every level of our being—physically, emotionally, psychologically, and spiritually. We grow into the next stage of our evolution and it happens almost effortlessly. Examples of this phenomenon appear regularly in our world today.

Suddenly, a talent for the piano emerges in a woman at the age of forty, who previously had no experience with the instrument. With regular practice and proper instruction, she is playing beautifully in a year. Another woman who has endured many years of abusive relationships suddenly frees herself from that pattern and finds dignity, self-love, and a healthy, rewarding relationship. A drug addict kicks his habit; an alcoholic overcomes his addiction; a person who has been seriously ill spontaneously is cured. We all know such people and have heard such stories many times over. The common thread implicit in all these experiences is that the transformation is made without extreme effort and, in every event, not by willpower alone. Conversely, there are many people in the very same circumstances who struggle valiantly but do not pick up instrument, or kick the habit, or overcome the pattern of abuse. What separates those who change from those who do not? What makes one set of people different from the other? In many cases, it is not effort. Indeed, those who struggle in vain often struggle harder than those who change.

Such profound transformations are made possible by a remarkable shift in the energetic patterns within the person's field. Something changed the field; we do not know who and we may not know how, but the field was changed and the person made some remarkable step that was previously believed to be impossible. This is not to say that such a change was without its emotional pain or suffering. Indeed, there is always some pain around letting go of an old pattern. But people who make these dramatic shifts invariably say that while they fought their addiction for decades, or struggled against their illness for years, the actual step was quite mysterious and remarkably easier than they had ever dreamed possible. No one can explain it, we say. It's a mystery, a miracle. Anyone who has witnessed the remarkable changes that occur in people when they release an old pattern from the field recognizes the process as miraculous.

Conversely, blockages in the energy field can restrict a person from making a step in evolution, even if the person wants desperately to make such a step and is doing everything he or she can think of to change.

Energetic Patterns and the False Self

Before I discuss how to make additional changes in the field, beyond those I discussed in chapter 8, let me talk about the kinds of patterns we have within us and which ones we need to release. All of the patterns that make up your life—whether they are genetic or environmental—can be grouped into two categories. The first set emerges from your true self, the inner being that you long to fully experience and express in the world. The second set makes up the false personality, which, when it is expressed, can sometimes give certain short-term pleasures but usually blocks the expression of your deeper self, and consequently leads into dark alleys, dead ends, and disappointments. You are the only person who can discern the difference between your true self and your false self, and the patterns each gives rise to. However, there is one test that can help you determine the source of a particular pattern: Behavior patterns that permit you to love yourself and others, promote self-expression, and give you deep connection to the source of life come from the true self and provide the deepest sense of happiness and satisfaction. Behavior patterns that arise out of chronic fears, anger, hostility, hatred, and feelings of dependency all emerge from delusion and the false self.

The false self prevents you from becoming happy and fulfilled because it does the two things that guarantee unhappiness. First, it prevents you from expressing your true nature, and second, at the same time, it blocks you from experiencing a deep and loving relationship with God, however you perceive Him/Her/It.

Patterns that obstruct the true self arise from one and only one cause: the training that love is conditional. To varying degrees all of us were raised on conditional love, meaning that we were loved or not loved according to our ability and willingness to conform to certain behaviors. Since our survival depended on that love, its tenuousness caused many of us to be shaken at the very roots of our being. Those who were raised on such an unstable love learned that reality always contains an implicit threat, and therefore requires a certain degree of conformity, adaptation, and sacrifice. The biggest sacrifice of all, of course, is the sacrifice of one's true nature, or simply one's true self.

People sacrifice that which they truly want to express because they believe that they cannot be themselves and at the same time be loved. Therefore, they must develop a way of being, a persona, that satisfies the people they depend on for love. That persona becomes the barrier that blocks us from experiencing the true self within. The persona is made up of many negative beliefs about ourselves, beliefs that can become powerful prisons.

A gifted dancer who believes she has insufficient ability, or none at all, may never realize her true talents and potential as a human being. That belief may well corrupt her life and cause endless suffering and sickness. Beliefs actually combine to form our personality—they describe how we think we should behave in given situations. They tell us what is possible and what isn't.

Such false or negative beliefs combine to form an outer personality that, like an ill-fitting costume, creates obstructions and energetic restrictions within this field. Negative beliefs are maintained in a vicious cycle, beginning with the repetition of that belief by the mind. Such statements as "I am no good" create wounds in the energetic field. Those wounds can become holes, or leaks, or they can be covered over by a kind of energetic scar tissue that forms blockages or boulders, thus blocking the flow of life force through your energy field. This creates eddies in one place, weak spots or tightnesses in others. Those blockages prevent the life force from flowing optimally to your cells, tissues, and organs. Leaks, blockages, and wounds in the field maintain negative thinking patterns and beliefs because they prevent fresh ideas from emerging in the field. In effect, the field is not as supple, changeable, and growing as it once was, and thus the life of old beliefs is sustained, which in turn sustains the wounds in the field.

Energetic Patterns Can Be the Cause of Disease

Once these energetic restrictions are imposed on your field, they manifest in the body as stress, muscle tension, restricted respiration, hormonal imbalances, and blocked blood and lymph flows. These energetic and physical conditions can become your accepted way of being. Gradually, they can affect your heartbeat and respiration, the amount of oxygen your tissues receive, the amount of carbon dioxide your body releases, the relative strength of your immune system, your posture, the way you move, the way you feel, and how you interact with others. In short, they can mold you into someone other than your true self, and in the process can make you ill.

Healing occurs when we break the circle by healing the wounds in the field and thus changing the energetic, physical, and psychological patterns. By removing the blockages in the energetic field, the life force flows abundantly to cells, organs, and even to the mind. Soon we feel better and see things differently. Old and negative beliefs are shed because we now begin to realize how capable and powerful we truly are.

Growing into health and maturity is, in effect, shedding those restrictive ideas that have been imposed on us. In a sense, it is an expansion of what we currently believe to be possible. It is a widening of consciousness or "expanded integrated awareness," which means that you expand your view of yourself so that those qualities that are implicit within you can emerge and express themselves.

As your innate qualities and talents emerge, you become aware of who you truly are. Your true nature steps out of the shadow of your unconscious and into the light of consciousness. Now you can begin to integrate your underlying abilities by creating a new, expanded picture of yourself. That's what I mean by expanded integrated awareness: It is the perception of the larger and truer you. Healing touch removes the barricades and opens the doors to your true self. Let me give an example.

Sam: Releasing Old Patterns

Sam is a thirty-eight-year-old man in a high-level, high-pressure, executive position. He came to me complaining of intense stress and stomach trouble. His day, he said, was essentially a race against time. He had too many appointments to make, too many deadlines to meet. He was very ambitious, but at the same time delicate: Anything and everything that went wrong in his world was perceived by Sam as evidence of his inadequacy or as a personal failure. He berated himself harshly. Yet, despite the fact that he was extremely hard on himself, or perhaps because of it, he continually strived to achieve more.

The physical side effects of such behavior were severe: chronic anxiety in the pit of his stomach, causing pain in his stomach and solar plexus, especially when he was under pressure. He also experienced pain whenever he missed a meal. Yet, he complained of chronic indigestion and took a lot of antacids. At the same time, he suffered from digestive problems, alternating between diarrhea and constipation. Stress impacts the human body in numerous ways, but I suspected that Sam might well have a congenital weakness in the gastrointestinal system, which is why his symptoms manifested there.

Sam's energetic patterning was clearly revealed by his nervous system's response to stress. The so-called flight-or-fight response is governed by the sympathetic nervous system, which shunts nerve innervation to the muscles and nerves in the heart, lungs, and periphery of the body whenever the body is under stress. This sends energy away from the digestive tract to the extremities so that the body can respond rapidly and aggressively in the face of danger.

Digestion, on the other hand, is conducted by the parasympathetic system, which directs nerve energy to the small and large intestines. Yet, Sam was continually under stress, and therefore under sympathetic dominance, which means that energy was continually being taken away from his digestive tract and channeled to his arms, legs, and cardiovascular system. Meanwhile, his stomach and third chakra would tighten, causing constriction of energy within the chakra and tightening of tissues and blood vessels within the organs. Sam often ate when he was stressed, which means that he was taking in food when there was insufficient nerve innervation and life force within the digestive tract. This causes digestion to be weakened and results in dyspepsia, bloating, gas, and putrefied food matter in the gut.

At the same time, stress tightens the diaphragm, causing the breathing to become shallow and emotional. Studies have shown that shallow breathing is associated with poorly oxygenated blood and cells, fatigue, weakness, and emotional instability. Not only did Sam suffer from all of these problems, but the chronic stress had brought on depression. He simply couldn't see himself carrying the burden any longer. Needless to say, Sam hated going to work in the morning.

After Sam told me of these issues, I immediately urged him to see a gastrointestinal specialist to determine if he suffered from an ulcer. In addition, I made numerous dietary recommendations, which Sam adopted, to support his stomach and digestive function.

Then I went to work on his field, focusing initially on the first, third, and fourth chakras. I tried to strengthen his first chakra in order to give him a stronger hold on the physical world and his own physical existence. Sam needed to feel grounded and centered, which the first chakra would give him. The third chakra needed to be strengthened to boost Sam's will, which had grown tired, weak, and frustrated. I channeled healing energy to the fourth chakra to boost his morale and overall emotional condition.

Clear the Spiritual Channel, or Central Tube, and Restore the Connection Between Heaven and Earth

In the last chapter, I showed how we can heal leaks and chakras to change the patterns within the field. Here, we want to take another step in changing patterns by removing blockages from the central tube, which is something I worked on with Sam.

As I pointed out in chapter 4, the central tube is a flow of energy that originates from a cosmic or heavenly source and runs from the top of the head to the base of the spine. It exits out of the spine and moves down into the earth. At the midpoint of this tube is the vibral core, and located along the tube are the seven chakras. The central tube is a shaft of energy, often referred to in other disciplines as the "spiritual channel," that is the energetic connection between the two great polarities of life: the infinite and the finite, heaven and earth. As such, the tube serves as the matrix around which the material body coalesces, and this is the channel through which life energy flows from the top of the body to the bottom.

The central tube can become clogged with old emotional debris, thus blocking one's sense of connection to the universe and the earth. The person with a blocked spiritual channel cannot feel an intuitive connection with the source of life, nor with Mother Earth. Without this feeling of connectedness, a person cannot draw inspiration from above or sustenance from below. One is neither a child of heaven nor a natural inhabitant of the earth. This is the ultimate experience of aloneness and isolation, and with such feelings comes a host of other negative emotions and attitudes toward life.

We can reestablish that sense of connection by clearing the central tube of obstructions. Once those obstructions are eliminated, a person begins to feel more relaxed in life. He feels more connected to his heavenly source, and therefore has greater faith in the forces that sustain him every day he exists. He can be inspired with ideas, creativity, and the power of the life energy that is streaming down upon each of us every instant of our lives. Not only that, but his connection with the earth is also improved, thus giving him a clearer sense of what must be done to secure his place on the earth. The physical, psychological, and spiritual effects of clearing the tube are profound and myriad, but they all add up to the same two great blessings: They improve our connection with the true self, and they reestablish our connection with the source of life.

Moving Old Energetic Waste Out of the Channel

Very often, when I am working with people like Sam, I finish my treatment by clearing the central tube. I do this form of treatment only after I have established a strong bond of trust because it requires the practitioner to touch the client's head, shoulders, and back. I have found that clearing the tube is highly effective at eliminating old emotional wounds, memories, and attachments to old relationships that limit the person's outlook and growth—even when the person doesn't even realize that he still holds on to such memories or relationships. It is also a powerful way to raise the life force. Keep in mind that clearing the tube is usually done at the end of a treatment. That means that by the time you clear the tube, you have centered, done your assessment, and finished your energy work. Here are the steps that you can use to clear your patient's central tube.

1. Move to the back of your patient and gently place your hands on the back of his neck with your thumbs gently pressing against the muscles on each side of the vertebrae at the base of the head. Massage these points ever so gently so that the muscles relax.

2. Slowly move your thumbs down the left and right sides of each vertebra, pausing at each vertebra to massage the muscles on each side of the spine. Do not stop until you reach the base of the spine.

3. Your intention in this first phase of the clearing is to loosen the muscles and gain the body's trust. The client may well trust you intellectually, but you must now convince his body that it can release its armor and allow you to probe its soft and vulnerable interior. Massage gently and firmly. You want your client to feel good, to relax, and to put down his armor so that you can go deeper with each step of the clearing.

4. Repeat the procedure again, moving from the top of the spine to its base, with the same loving, healing hands.

5. Do the procedure a third time. As you move down the spine this time, go a little deeper. Try to wake up the spinal nerves so that energy is released into the system.

6. Begin again from the top vertebra, only this time move your own life force beyond your hands, so that your "etheric hands" move deeply into the client's inner field and directly into the central tube running through the center of the body. Your energetic hands are now deep within the tube and you can sense where the blockages in the tube are located. Merely

loosen the blockages that you sense and then keep moving downward through the tube. Allow yourself to perceive any information your client's field may be communicating to you about these blockages, but more important, stay focused on your work, stay centered, and keep reciting your prayer (if that is the tool you use to keep yourself centered).

7. When you reach the base of the spine, keep your thumbs at the base and rest your hands on the sides of each buttock. Between your hands, create an energy ball. Visualize the energy forming and becoming stronger and more vital at the base of the client's spine. You are now strengthening the client's Qi, or life force. Take a few minutes and allow the energy ball to grow and become strong.

8. When you feel the ball is strong enough and of very good quality Qi, slowly begin to move your thumbs up on either side of the vertebrae while visualizing the energy gently moving with your hands. As the energy moves upward, it serves as a vacuum cleaner, gathering all the old blockages and debris from the tube.

9. As you reach the back of the client's heart chakra, pause and ask the client to take a deep breath. With his inhalation, continue moving up the spine to the base of the head. Try to visualize and "feel" the ball growing ever more powerful as you move up the spine.

10. At the base of the neck, gently place your hands and palms on either side of the client's head. Ask him to exhale and to visualize the release of all he no longer needs out of the top of his head. At the same time, gently squeeze his head between your hands and pull the ball of energy and debris that it holds out of the top of his central tube at the top of his head.

11. As you raise your hands high above your client's head, release the debris into the Light of Love, to be transformed by the Great Healer.

    If the client feels congestion in his neck, repeat the process from step 6 to the end.

Many people describe the feeling upon being released from central tube debris as an "energy rush." Others feel lighter, and still others feel tired and need to rest for a while.

Using Energy to Change—Sam's Story Continues

Sam continued to see me once a week or twice a month for about six months as I worked on his central tube. During this period, we made gradual but steady progress. The central issue, as far as my practice was concerned, was getting Sam to see life in different terms, which is to say, to see life in a more positive light. Sam believed too strongly in the delusion that he had to be responsible for every little detail in his personal and professional life. He was assuming way too much responsibility in every situation. Underlying this attitude was his hidden belief that everything goes wrong in life, that the universe is an unfriendly and even a hostile place, and that every weak link in the chain of life will be broken. It was up to Sam to make the links strong, he secretly contended. This belief was very strong in him. It didn't matter to Sam when I told him that every link in the chain of life is weak and that every day is filled with millions of tenuous dramas that were all going in his favor even though he was unwilling or unable to see these positive events. It didn't matter when I said that each and every time he experienced a difficult day at work, or believed that a project was about to fail, he had, in fact, had a successful day and the project he was working on would succeed. It didn't matter a bit to him when I told him that he was a successful man and that he was high up in the corporate world in which he lived. All of this only served to reinforce his belief that he had to go on struggling to succeed. "Sam, you are where you are in spite of your struggle," I said.

These words, of course, were meaningless against the powerful energetic pattern that existed within him. Sam and I could have gone back into his past and analyzed all the details of his childhood. That may or may not have changed things. Given the fact that so many people undergo therapy today, and so few actually emerge from their patterns, I suspected that therapy alone would not be adequate to change Sam. (Although it is my experience that psychotherapy works very well in conjunction with healing touch.) What existed at the bottom of his belief system was, in all likelihood, a very powerful energetic pattern comprised of emotional scar tissue and blockages that prevented the transformative energy of heaven and earth from changing his life. He could not get adequate life force to evolve, to change, and to let go of the energetic debris that was holding him back. And in order to do that, we would have to eliminate the blockages in his field and his tube.

I tried to do this every time we got together. I especially concentrated on Sam's tube. I perceived that Sam's tube was heavily scarred. As I removed the scar tissue and blockages from Sam's field and central tube, Sam began to have insights about his relationship with his father, who regularly undermined him as a child and prevented him from ever feeling truly safe in his family. Sam realized that the central power in his life, his father, was hostile to him, which had conditioned him to believe that the power in life was negative. When he began to consider all the ramifications of this conditioning, Sam began to refer to his father's behavior as a kind of "emotional and spiritual abuse."

Meanwhile, Sam began to realize that his adult life was remarkably successful, despite the problems of his childhood. This stood in stark contrast to his childhood, which triggered another round of revelations in Sam about the possible nature of reality and about his relationship with God. Many things were going right in his life, Sam realized, though in the past he had been afraid to acknowledge them. He had prevented himself from appreciating his blessings, he said, because he feared exposing them to the hostile universe, which he believed would wipe out the good in his life if that good was ever exposed by Sam's open appreciation. This caused Sam to focus exclusively on his problems, which gave him an internal life of strife and, in turn, began to destroy his health.

The miracle of Sam's transformation was that while he

changed no lights flashed on and no fireworks went off. One day, he confessed to me: "I'm starting to feel better about things. I'm actually enjoying my work more," he said. "I think I'm changing." Gradually, Sam's outlook on life did change, and with this change his stomach and digestive disorders disappeared. I would say that healing touch helped Sam to accept life; it also helped him open up to the reality that he was being supported a lot more than he had previously believed or was willing to admit. He became a much more positive person, especially in his feelings toward himself, yet there was no one instance or single moment that he could point to and say, That's when I changed for the better.

After many of my sessions with Sam, I would lead him through a visualization I call the rainbow meditation, which is designed to help us overcome whatever beliefs may be holding us back or keeping us in fear, scarcity, and old patterns.

EXERCISE: RAINBOW MEDITATION FOR PLENTY

1. Visualize above your head a disk of utterly beautiful and vibrant rainbow light. This rainbow disk represents the opening into "the spiritual field of plenty." It is a ring of energy, an opening into the abundance that has been provided for your soul in this life. Within this ring, all that you need is available to you. Visualize the disk open and available to you now.

2. Reach up with your hands and see yourself pulling down from this spiritual realm all that you need, no matter whether that need be material, psychological, or spiritual—or all three (see diagram 10).

3. This visualization can be done at any time, but the intention may vary depending on when it is done. If you do this exercise upon awakening, try to visualize bringing down through your whole body all that you need to promote healing on the physical, emotional, mental, and spiritual levels. Also, visualize receiving through the disk of rainbow light whatever help you need that day.

DIAGRAM 10. RAINBOW DISK

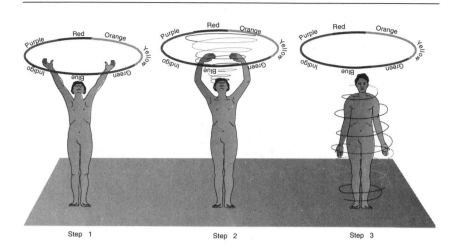

Step 1   Step 2   Step 3

If you are performing the meditation to help you serve a patient better, do it silently after you center yourself and before you do your prayer. In this case, visualize yourself bringing down through the circle of light all that the recipient needs to be healed. Do the meditation as you stand behind the recipient, very close to her back.

If you are leading a friend, loved one, or client through the meditation, do it at the conclusion of the session and ask the person to silently visualize herself receiving all that she needs through the circle of rainbow light. Before you do the meditation, go to the back of the person and stand close to it. Visualize the disk above the recipient's head. See the recipient reach up into the disk to bring down with her hands all that she needs for her complete healing. And always end this session with a prayer of thanksgiving for all that is being healed.

Healing Yourself to Know Yourself

Knowing the true self is perhaps our greatest goal, for in coming to know ourselves we come to understand our relationship to the universe at large. In that knowing is the realization that each of us is loved—indeed, that we are loved far more than we can conceive of. This invariably is the perception people experience when they go beyond their conditioning. Reaching beyond our conditioning isn't easy, however. Very often it feels as if we are hitting a wall, and indeed we are—it is a wall of energy that must be healed. For the practitioner of healing touch, psychological conditioning is not some abstract term that is applied to behavior patterns but is an energetic fact, a blockage, that prevents change from occurring smoothly and relatively painlessly. Energetic patterns and blockages cause us pain, and that pain is real. The reason is simple: Change is a constant; the universe demands evolution and transformation. This is both the fact and the fabric of life. But if we are blocked, we cannot move with the universal rhythms, and therefore we cannot see the light toward which we all are traveling.

A Healer's Checklist

Here is a step-by-step snapshot of your healing session—a checklist, so to speak. Use this list as an overview to help guide you through a session.

1. Have the patient sit on a stool or a straight-backed chair with the back and front and right sides exposed.
2. Ask the patient to do the "flowing water" visualization, along with deep breathing into the bottom of the stomach.
3. Assume your position behind the patient, with your left hand raised (palm up) and your right hand lowered (palm facing the earth). Center yourself.
4. Begin saying your prayer.
5. "Turn on your hands" by rubbing them vigorously and then creating the energy ball between your hands. Pass the energy ball into the person's field.
6. Do your initial assessment.

7.   Open the feet so that the life force flows through to the earth.

8.   Clear the field and chakras of restrictions, tension, blockages, and boulders.

9.   Close the holes in the field.

10. Balance the excessive and deficient areas.

11. Release all energy that you remove from the field into the Light of Love.

12. Do a second assessment.

13. Check the feet again to assure that the energy is flowing out from them.

14. Clear the tube by moving the energy up the spine and pulling it off the top of the head.

15. When the main part of the treatment is finished, return to your standing position, with your hands over your solar plexus, restoring yourself to peace and harmony.

16. Have the patient lie down.

17. Balance the chakras.

18. Allow the patient ten minutes to rest and integrate the treatment.

10

Working with Specific Illnesses and Serious Disease

Healing touch can be used in conjunction with all other therapies to treat any illness. No matter what the disease, your primary focus is to restore the optimal flow of life energy through the field. You will be doing this by clearing away blockages in the field, closing the holes and leaks, moving excessive energy to the areas of the field that are deficient, channeling additional life force to places that are weak, clearing and balancing the chakras, and clearing the central tube. While you are doing this, you remain centered. Whenever necessary, you enhance the flow of energy within the client, and between the two of you, by using the meditations and guided images I have provided. This is your work, no matter what the disharmony with which your client may be working.

Nevertheless, it's essential that you tailor your treatment to the specific imbalances you may be facing. Following is a set of guidelines for dealing with specific illnesses that you may face in your practice. These recommendations can be used by anyone who wishes to use healing touch to help a friend or family member. As I said in chapter 3, treatment time varies according to the severity of the illness. There are times when very short sessions are all that should be done, and there are other times when you can take a longer period to work on the client's field.

How do you decide the correct work? Let's go through some examples.

Colds and Flu

Healing touch is very helpful in the treatment of acute illnesses such as the common cold and flu. It helps to alleviate many of the symptoms by decongesting and clearing the energy field. It also speeds the healing process.

The traditional view of the common cold is very different from the one we typically hold in the modern, Western culture. Traditionally, colds were considered the body's method of housecleaning—that is, of eliminating accumulating waste, toxins, bacteria, viruses, and stagnant energy. Sneezing, coughing, runny nose, diarrhea, and frequent urination are all the body's attempts to discharge these toxins rapidly and efficiently. As the study of immunology has proven, fever is a deliberate act of the immune system (namely, CD4 cells and macrophages) to create a hostile environment against pathogens. In other words, it is all part of the body's attempt to heal itself. In this view, the symptoms of the cold actually serve a very positive purpose and should be allowed to do their work. Suppressing the symptoms of a cold with various pharmaceuticals—the customary approach to colds in our modern culture—prevents the body from cleansing itself.

But cleansing is only one aspect of the cold's job. Traditional healers have viewed the cold and flu as the body's demand for rest. Many healers also view a cold as a release of old and unexpressed emotions, especially sadness and grief. In other words, it can be thought of as a safety valve, a long cry, particularly when we have neglected our emotional lives.

Whenever you work on a person with a cold or flu, work on the sixth chakra (sinuses), the fifth chakra (the throat and ears), the fourth chakra (the heart, especially to strengthen one's emotional life and assist in the release of emotions), and the second chakra (to promote elimination through the intestines).

Do your assessment in all of these areas. Usually, you will discover feelings of "thickness" and/or "heat" in one or more of these areas, indicating congestion and increased blood flow. Generally, you will spiral the energy out of the second, fourth, fifth, and sixth chakra areas. To do this, enter the chakra by moving your hand slowly in a counterclockwise direction, cup your hand, and lift stagnant energy out of the chakra. Do this for all the chakras that are involved in the cold symptoms. Pay particular attention to the chakras that are congested, such as the sinuses (sixth chakra), or the bowels (second chakra), if the client is constipated. Once that is done, open the secondary chakras on the feet. This will allow excess energy to be discharged from the body and new, healing earth's energy to enter the body. Again, it is better to begin at the bottom of the tube and work your way up.

Healing touch will boost the healing forces within the body and speed up the elimination and healing process, thus helping the client avoid an unnecessarily long cold. Keep the treatment short: no more than ten minutes.

If you perform the work for a longer period, it could trigger an even bigger discharge and cause a very intense discharge over a twenty-four- to forty-eight-hour period.

A friend of mine worked on one of the doctors in our office who had just begun to experience mild cold symptoms. In her attempt to do a good and thorough energy treatment, she spent about twenty minutes doing healing touch. When the doctor got home that night, he developed a fever of 103 degrees and was in bed with severe symptoms for two straight days. My friend might well have done him a great service, because this forced him to rest and allowed his body to eliminate a lot of accumulated waste, but the suffering was excessive, as far as he was concerned, and could have been avoided had she worked on him consistently for shorter periods of time. This would have allowed the elimination to be gradual and painless, while she strengthened the healing energies in his field.

Usually, seven to ten minutes of healing touch are all you need to help alleviate the symptoms of a cold and enhance the body's own healing forces.

Remember, the physical body is the densest part of the field. Disharmony occurs in the energetic body before it manifests in the physical. The physical body is the final discharge point in a process that begins in the field and finally manifests in the body. All energetic disturbances start the disease process by affecting the body on a cellular level. If the cell wall is compromised, there can then be bacterial or viral invasion of the cell, creating a virulent cold. However, if blockages, stagnation, and destabilizing energy can be eliminated from the field, the cells can be protected and the virus or bacteria cannot gain a foothold in the system. By reducing the disturbance in the field, you will reduce the harmful energetic forces and thus reduce the symptoms of the illness. Even if a virus or bacteria is taken in, the symptoms may only be mild, such as a little nasal discharge, but no significant disease process will develop.

In addition to energy work, the patient should get plenty of rest and take in adequate fluids, especially if there is fever. If the symptoms worsen considerably or persist longer than one week, you may need to encourage him or her to see a medical doctor.

When Treating Fever, Reduce the Energy

A fever occurs when tissues are injured from one or another of several possible causes, among them: some type of invasive event such as surgery or a blow to the body; a vascular accident, such as a heart attack; an infection caused by a virus, bacteria, or protozoa; diseases that trigger an autoimmune response such as arthritis; or certain types of cancers.

Once tissues are injured, the immune system sends out a signal to raise the body's temperature to prevent bacteria or viruses from gaining a foothold in the injured tissues. The fever itself is triggered by CD4 cells, the commander or general of the immune system. These cells send out orders to the rest of the immune system by producing powerful chemical messengers, collectively known as cytokines. These cytokines, in turn, trigger a battery of changes in your body, including a rise in the body's temperature, creating inflammation (which increases heat and blood flow to the affected area), and signals to your brain to make you sleepy. Once you're resting, your immune system can direct your body's energy to fight the injury or pathogen.

Thus, fever is part of the body's healing mechanism. In general, most physicians will tell a person not to treat a fever unless it gets beyond 104 degrees Fahrenheit.

Unlike pharmaceuticals, which will suppress the fever and thus deprive the body of its good work, healing touch strengthens the healing forces within the body and thus reduces the need for a high fever. Healing touch will also bring down a fever by reducing the destabilizing energies within the field.

One of the many ironies of the body's healing mechanisms is that while inflammation is produced by the body in its efforts to heal, the swelling that accompanies inflammation gets in the way of healing by blocking blood flow. Sometimes the swelling is so severe that the flows of energy and blood are blocked or severely restricted. There is also a heat reaction throughout the body as a result of the injury. Invariably, you will feel heat and congested energy in the field over areas of inflammation.

Treat fever and inflammation by removing the heat and congested energy from the field with your hands. Then build an energy ball within the vibral core and visualize the area surrounded by the color dark blue. The dark blue color cools the body and has an antiinflammatory effect. Your hands may become very hot. This means you are removing the heat from the body.

As the temperature begins to decrease in your hands, visualize the color of the light in the energy ball becoming green, which has a balancing effect on the area.

Do not send life force into the body initially. This will serve to further inflame the condition. Do this only as the patient becomes stronger. The treatment time should be one to five minutes initially and gradually increase to ten to twelve minutes.

Unblocking the Field to Alleviate Headaches

In general, headaches are caused by congestion or constricted energy in the lower chakras, which block life force from flowing out of the feet. Instead, the energy backs up into the head and causes a headache.

These treatments can last anywhere from five to fifteen minutes and consist mainly of opening the root chakra and the secondary chakras at the bottoms of the feet so that the backed-up energy in the head can drain. In cases like this, we move to the opposite end of the pain.

The primary work is to open the feet and clear the constriction most often found in the area of the solar plexus. The feet may have to be held for up to five minutes at a time. Ask the client to take deep breaths into the bottoms of her feet as you conduct the work. The deep breathing will help release the diaphragm and open the solar plexus area as well.

Also, remove blockages in the chakra at the solar plexus. Clear the shoulders of any tension and gently massage the neck and shoulders to loosen the throat chakra area. The massage here is similar to the massaging of the legs and feet required for opening the feet. With a headache there is usually tension in the shoulder and a palpable tightness. A gentle massage here will stimulate energy flow. You can then proceed with the regular energy work around the body. If the headache is of a sinus nature, clear any congestion found in the second chakra (sacral) as well (see the section on the chakra energy spiral in chapter 5).

The headache will usually ease, if not disappear completely, during the treatment. Encourage the client to go home and rest for an hour or so. If the headache is not gone at the end of the treatment, resting afterward will probably take care of the headache completely.

The life energy can be boosted if the shoulders relax during treatment and if the headache is not severe. If the life energy is raised during a severe headache with very tight shoulder muscles, it will only exacerbate the headache. Severe headaches (especially migraines) need supportive, gentle treatment, especially in the early sessions with your client.

Catastrophic Disease: Make the Treatments Short

In general, when treating catastrophic illnesses such as cancer or AIDS, less is more. The sicker the patient, the less you treat. Very sick patients can be treated for short periods (up to five minutes) every day. The treatment consists of clearing and balancing the energy field. My experience is that very sick clients are extremely appreciative of healing touch because of its effects on fatigue and because it calms and often balances the chaotic, destabilizing, and destructive influences within the field. These energies cause the rapid progression of the disease and create a sense of instability within the client. Practitioners have also noted that clients experience better rest and often require less pain medication with regular healing touch treatments.

When the patient is very ill and is unable to sit up, do not raise the life energy. Since catastrophic illness depletes the Qi, trying to raise it in the very ill patient can cause more pain and most certainly more energy depletion.

When treating people with cancer, *do not send energy to the area of the tumor.* This will only serve to strengthen the disease and make it more virulent. Instead, the work should focus on supporting healthy tissue and maintaining its health and integrity. The stronger and healthier the unaffected tissue, the less likely it will be to be invaded by the disease. Focus your energy work on the healthy tissue to make it so strong that it can resist the assault of the un-healthy cells, and thus prevent the illness from spreading.

Julie's Story

Julie began seeing me in July 1988 at age forty. Eight and a half years earlier, she had been diagnosed with ovarian cancer and had a radical hysterectomy. She also underwent radiation treatment, chemotherapy and another pelvic operation that resulted in a co-lostomy. Her presenting complaints at the time of her first visit were incomplete digestion and difficulty in wearing her colostomy appliance without developing irritation and polyps around the opening, or stoma. She had also developed a considerable amount of scar tissue in the abdominal area. Scar tissue impairs energy flow within the field and the physical body.

Since I am also a nutritionist, my initial work with Julie was to give her dietary advice. The digestive system and stoma had to be stabilized before she could trust me to give her energy work. As Julie put it, "I felt my body wasn't receptive to anything until I could receive food."

Nine months after we began working on the physical body, or the "root" of the energy field, she was digesting her food well, feel-ing more energetic for activities of daily living, and was less de-pressed. She also was wearing her colostomy appliance for three days between changes with no irritation around the stoma.

We began energy work with a meditation to make her sensi-tive to the way energy moves in the body. The guided imagery helped Julie reconnect to the organs that she had lost to surgery, but were still there as energetic organs in the etheric field (see chapter 4 to refresh your knowledge of the etheric field). We then started healing touch, initially focusing on integrating and releasing the emotions related to the loss of her female organs. We did energy work for nine months, during which time Julie made remarkable progress in integrating very difficult emotions and restoring her sense of femininity.

After this period, Julie and I began to work on the scar tissue within her stoma and intestinal tract. We were joined in this work by an acupuncturist whose specialty is eliminating scar tissue. The three of us worked together for the next two years. At one point, her surgeon, who examined Julie periodically, reported how amazed he was that the scar tissue in her abdomen had decreased so markedly. In fact, Julie had made so much healing progress that her surgeon said that he would consider reversing the colostomy in the future if she continued to make such progress.

Julie's critique of her four-year process of energy work is as follows:

"Energy work lightens up the physical body. It seems to release physical blocks to feelings. As the parts of my body released, I felt more available to spirit. I began to be more able to trust the movement and changes in life. Initially, I saw myself as having very separate parts. My mind was very separate from my heart, which was very separate from my stomach and intestines and other organs. Energy work has helped me see and feel myself as a whole being—an integration of body, mind, and spirit.

"It has also helped me gain a trust of living.

"As I've become more conscious of having to breathe during energy work, I feel more empowered and in control. I feel like I am participating in the healing effort, which also makes me feel less of a victim. As I have surrendered to the process, I am owning more of my intuitive and spiritual self."

Working with Terminal Illness: Giving Peace and Comfort in Life's Most Challenging Hour

Facing death is hard enough, but facing it alone is a tragedy beyond words. When working with a client who is clearly terminal, your work is intended to assist the spirit as it prepares to leave the physical form. You are there to make the transition easier and to contribute to the loving, spiritual, and gentle forces that are now at work in the client's life. Healing touch offers the gentle power of love, and that is what a person needs most when making life's most frightening transition. The practice can help relax the client's body and clarify his mind, open his chakras, and assist his birth process into the next world. The healing energy you give to the client will assist him in many ways—physically, emotionally, psychologically, and spiritually. But the very fact that this is energetic healing, that you are addressing the spirit and not the body, is crucial to the person who is dying. Your presence and your work are a statement of love and faith: There is more to this life than the body you are about to leave.

The actual energy work usually lasts for only five minutes.

During the dying process, as the spirit prepares to vacate the earthly body, the lower three chakras begin to lose their integrity. The spirit, or soul, is no longer firmly rooted in the body. The patient is not always coherent and may appear to lie talking with someone who is not physically in the room. When this is occurring, one does not try to "ground" the patient by holding his feet and directing energy downward. Instead, calm and smooth the field; groom it, so to speak, by running your hands slowly and gently over the front of the body (if the client is in bed and lying on his back) or the sides of the body, whichever is available to you. Try to remove any blockages that may be holding the spirit back or causing pain or suffering. When you've done this, open the crown chakra. To do that, hold your hands just above the head at the seventh chakra and send gentle energy upward. This chakra is actually a great circle of energy above the head. It is now drawing the life energy out of the body and collecting it unto itself as it prepares to return to its natural home, the world of spirit. Visualize the chakra opening and the spirit being able to release itself from the body whenever it chooses to do so. You are only assisting in the process that the spiritual world has well in hand.

The energy work helps calm and relax the patient and allows for an easier transition. It is important to remember that healing touch cannot cause or speed death. Death is a private process between the individual and the Creator.

Crystal's Story

Crystal, a forty-two-year-old woman suffering from acute myelocytic leukemia, wanted me to do energy work with her in preparation for a bone marrow transplant. She had been diagnosed with leukemia two years earlier and had since tried some nontraditional approaches. This alternative treatment had kept her in remission for two years, but the leukemia had become active again. Since she had a bone marrow donor, she decided to go the more orthodox route while incorporating healing touch.

I worked with Crystal every two to three days over a two-month period. During this time, Crystal fought a life-threatening fungal sinus infection and underwent intensive chemotherapy and antibiotic therapy in preparation for the bone marrow transplant.

During the eight weeks, my focus with Crystal was to help her center herself and strengthen her own inherent healing abilities. She showed remarkable courage and stamina in dealing with the side effects of chemotherapy and the disappointment that her body was not able to handle the treatments that would prepare her for the transplant. If she could not respond to the chemotherapy there could be no transplant.

Often I would work on her liver. After smoothing her field and attempting to balance her central tube, I would hold my hands over her liver (front and back) and build a healing ball of energy between them, concentrating on the liver. I did this to support her liver as it tried to deal with the toxic pharmaceuticals being introduced into her body. These treatments would last seven to ten minutes.

Many of the nurses and doctors were very skeptical of healing touch at first, and some were openly critical. They argued that she was going to die and she should not have tried nonorthodox approaches in the first place. Meanwhile, Crystal was improving. She felt better and had significantly more vitality after I conducted each treatment. Her physicians and nurses could not help but notice, and they were remarkably forthcoming with me in their support. "I don't know what you're doing, but she feels better and is less agitated after you've worked with her," one doctor told me. "Keep doing it." They also reported that she rested easier and was not as nauseous after the treatments.

It soon became apparent, however, that all I could do was make her comfortable. She was losing her battle against the leukemia, and the highly toxic drugs she was being given were far too powerful. She returned to her home to be with her family. I visited her a couple of times very near to the end of her life. The healing touch took on a very different tenor at this stage. The treatments were three to four minutes in length and consisted of smoothing the field, clearing any debris in the lower three chakras, opening the crown chakra, and preparing the path for the spirit to exit the body. Although Crystal died, she made her passing gently and with great dignity.

Her husband shared his perception of the healing touch process as he watched it unfold:

"Healing touch helped Crystal focus her own innate healing powers. While it is easy for someone to say that Crystal died, and therefore all treatment was a failure, that was not the case. She came back against astronomical odds to beat a deadly fungal infection. While we will never know exactly how she came back, in my own mind, it was some blend of her astounding will, the intravenous medicine, and the energy work.

"Into the insane, hectic medical model of a cancer hospital setting, the healer and energy work brought a sense of safe space and trusting. Crystal believed in this work and resonated with it. There was a magical sense when you [Deby] came into her room. I would shut the door and protect the room from intrusion. Then you and Crystal would do your work.

"There was a deep consistency in the work, although it varied according to Crystal's physical condition, her mental condition, and the healer's inner sense of what was appropriate. Crystal always felt safe and that it helped her."

A Dynamic Treatment Plan

A good treatment plan always begins with a good initial interview. The healer should take a complete health history of the client as well as the presenting complaints. An extended family history should be obtained, along with information on any medicines, herbs, or vitamins or dietary supplements the patient is currently taking. It is also imperative that the healer have a working knowledge of the disease or disharmony the patient wants to work on. Invest in a few good textbooks on internal medicine, such as a *Merck Manual, Taber's Cyclopedic Medical Dictionary,* or *Harrison's Principles of Internal Medicine.*

Once you have established what the client sees as a problem, a care plan can be developed to guide both you and the patient through the treatment.

There is a five-step process that takes into consideration the patient's medical diagnosis and leads the healer to develop a plan of action to enhance the healing of the patient. The steps are as follows:

1. Assessment: This includes all information obtained in the initial interview.
2. Analysis: This includes analysis of the patient's problems.
3. Plan: In healing touch, the plan is the energy work, based on prioritizing the problems and establishing patient-centered goals, along with the specific intervention and rationale. This also includes the networking and the list of other professionals involved on the care team. The plan of energy work remains the same. What changes each week are the symptoms the patient arrives with and the changes that have occurred in the field as a result of the past week's work. Part of the plan is to talk with the patient and help him recognize the changes and evaluate the effect the work is having on him.
4. Implementation: This is putting the care plan into action to fulfill the patient-centered goals.

5. Evaluation: This includes determining the value and results of the treatment plan and evaluating the patient's progress. The evaluation comes from the patient, the family, other health care professionals involved (psychotherapist, massage therapist, chiropractor, family doctor, other nurse practitioners, etc.), and most important, from the healer observing the patient's response to the therapeutic touch process.

When a patient comes to you for healing touch, it is very important that he or she has had a recent physical examination by a doctor and that you are aware of any physical problems or limitations the patient may have.

For example, it was imperative that Sam (chapter 9) see a gastrointestinal specialist to rule out any type of ulcerative condition. If Sam had developed a bleeding ulcer, the first step in the care plan would be to stop the bleeding, not to do energy work on his solar plexus! Energy work may be appropriate, as are counseling on stress reduction and proper diet, but only after the life-threatening condition is identified and stabilized.

With certain conditions and illnesses, alternative health care methods work very well. However, if the patient finds himself facing a life-threatening situation, such as bleeding ulcers, extreme labile blood pressure, certain advanced stages of cancer, even broken bones, it is necessary to seek allopathic or orthodox medical treatment—in addition to doing healing touch. This brings us to the planning stages of our treatment phase, which includes the use of other caregivers in the healing process. If your client faces acute emotional issues and you are not qualified to handle them in a proper manner, your responsibility is to encourage the client to find a psychotherapist or therapeutic group situation to help him deal with the issues the two of you are uncovering with energy work.

Keeping in mind the importance of proper referral for physical and emotional needs, know that there are many other methods of healing that may enhance the treatment. For example, acupuncture and Chinese medicine may be helpful for the patient. They also enhance the energy work. Other good compatible modalities include massage, physical therapy, chiropractic, homeopathy, and nutritional counseling. Sometimes combining therapies helps move the patient toward health at a faster, more comfortable rate.

Five minutes of healing touch before any kind of massage or body work can make the body work session much more healing. By the same token, five minutes of energy work prior to a psychotherapy session can also enhance the work and productivity of the session.

Although treatment plans or care plans have been traditionally used in nursing, they can be modified for psychotherapy and body work.

The treatment plan is dynamic and does not remain static. It changes and expands as the energy needs of the patient change. The energy work creates the need for the dynamic treatment plan. The therapeutic touch and energy work usually help the patient to move and release at a faster but still safe pace. Therefore, each week you may find that different areas in the central tube need attention and support based on the healing that resulted from the work you and the patient did the prior week. Dynamic treatment comes with the healer's ability to implement treatment based on the growth and changes occurring within the patient.

Conclusion: Recognizing Spirit as the Healer

We are living in a time when the old duality that separates body and mind, energy and matter, is giving way. Quantum physics is teaching us that at the molecular level, scientists cannot determine whether matter is composed of particles or waves of energy. In fact, physicists tell us that the central factor that determines the essential nature of reality—that is, whether matter is made up of tiny bits of substance or waves of energy—is the mind. Look at the material world one way and you see particles as the basis of life; look at the matter in another way and you see waves. The only conclusion to be drawn is that reality is composed of both matter and energy, particles *and* waves.

We practitioners of healing touch couldn't agree more. We wish to point out, however, that for too long our society has stressed the material aspects of life, while it has undervalued the energetic or spiritual part of our being. Each of us is matter and energy, body and soul.

Science is now making the most tenuous of forays into the realm of energy and is coming up with many surprising discoveries that support the age-old view of human existence. Naturally, this frightens many people. It shakes our worldview at its very foundation. To think that you could affect someone at a distance with your thoughts, or that you could use your hands to send healing energy to someone you care about—these ideas run counter to many of our society's most fundamental beliefs. We take it for granted that, while we might have been raised in a very religious home, we base our belief system on materialistic ideas. The materialistic view of life maintains that you are your body and that's all you are. Not only is that a sad and frightening idea, but it is so limiting. Those who embrace this materialistic worldview ultimately discover that it leads to a very dark and lonely dead end.

Fortunately for all of us—including the disbelievers—we are much more than matter. We are energy, too. What we have only begun to discover—or, I should say, rediscover—is that there is tremendous power in the realization that we are luminous beings, living spheres of energy, who possess the ability to share that living energy with one another. For practitioners of healing touch, that means utilizing this practice as a tool against all types of disharmonies, including those that threaten life.

For those just starting out as practitioners, that means walking into difficult situations and employing the work even before you have sufficient experience to know as a certainty how powerful the practice really is—even before you know in your heart that matter is composed of both particles and waves and that you can transmit those waves of energy to another human being to make a profound difference in his or her life. Those of us who have been around a while and who have had that experience, have the joy and the comforting knowledge that there is more to life than merely the particles that make up the body.

In the end, healing touch is a challenge to the most fundamental beliefs of our society, to our modern world, and to each of us. Yet, it is the most liberating of practices and among the most powerful because it puts you in harmony with a greater reality, one that has sustained the world from the very beginning and will go on sustaining it forever.

Appendix 1

Intake Questionnaire

DATE   /   /

PATIENT

HOME ADDRESS

CITY   STATE   ZIP

HOME PHONE   WORK PHONE

OCCUPATION

MARITAL STATUS   AGE   BIRTHDATE

REFFERED BY

PRESENT AILMENT/SYMPTOMS

FAMILY HISTORY: FATHER:

MOTHER: SIBLINGS:

FAMILY HEALTH HISTORY: ARITHITIS   CANCER

HIGH BLOOD PRESSURE   DIABETES   TB

ASTHMA   GOITER   MENTAL

HEART DISEASE   GOUT   OBESITY

KIDNEY _____ EPILEPSY _____ ALLERGIES _____

OTHER _____

PERSONAL HEALTH HISTORY: TB _____ SCARLET FEVER _____ PNEUMONIA _____

INFECTIOUS DISEASES (i.e. measles, chicken pox, mumps) _____

TONSILLITIS _____ HEART DISEASE _____ HYPERTENSION _____

VENEREAL DISEASE _____

OTHER _____

_____

_____

_____

_____

LIST ALL SURGERIES: _____

_____

_____

_____

HABITS: LIST NORMAL BREAKFAST, LUNCH, DINNER FOR YOURSELF _____

BREAKFAST _____

LUNCH _____

DINNER _____

HOW MUCH/HOW OFTEN? _____

ALCOHOL _____ TOBACCO _____ DRUGS _____ COFFEE _____ TEA _____

WATER _____ SLEEP _____ BOWEL HABITS _____ EXERCISE _____

LIST ALL MEDICATIONS, VITAMINS, OR HERBS YOU ARE CURRENTLY TAKING

_____

_____

_____

FEMALE MENSTRUAL HISTORY: CYCLE ONSET _____ PERIODICITY _____

DURATION _____ TYPE OF FLOW: HEAVY MEDIUM LIGHT PAIN

COLOR: BRIGHT RED _____ DARK RED _____ CLOTS _____ MOOD SWINGS

BREAST TENDERNESS _____ WATER RETENTION _____ LAST MENSTRUAL PERIOD

OTHER _____

PREGNANCIES: CHILDREN _____ MISCARRIAGES _____ ABORTIONS

BIRTH CONTROL _____ D&C _____

COMMENTS YOU WISH TO MAKE: _____

_____

_____

SIGNED: _____

Appendix 2

Energy Work Treatment with the Patient in the Sitting Position

1

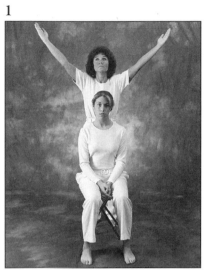

2

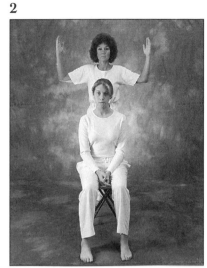

1-2: Practitioner opening Rainbow Disk and pulling energy down to herself.

3

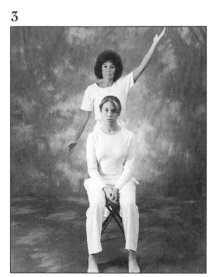

4

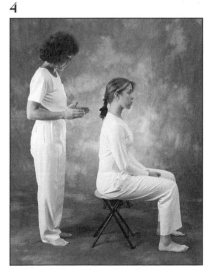

3: Practitioner collecting energy for the energy ball.

4: Practitioner forming the energy ball.

5

6

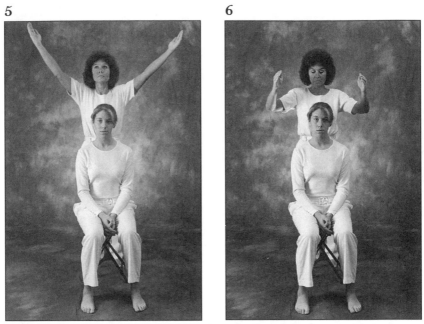

5-6: Practitioner opening Rainbow Disk and pulling down energy for the patient.

7

8

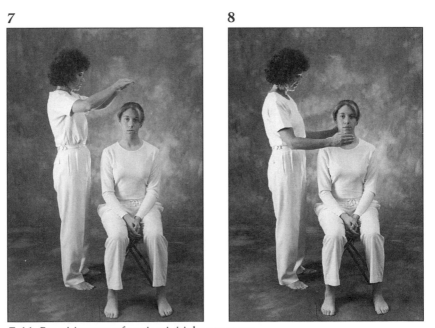

7-11: Practitioner performing initial assessment.

9

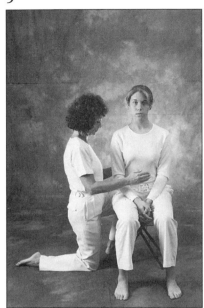

10

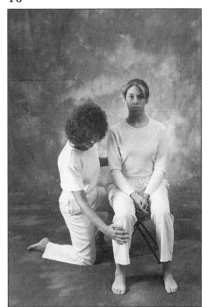

11

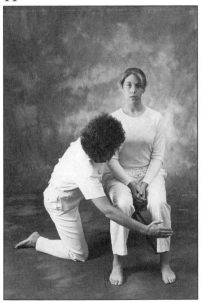

12   **13**

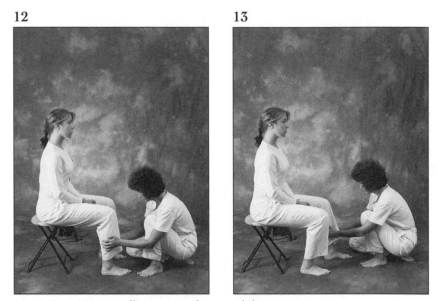

12-13: Practitioner pulling energy down each leg.

14

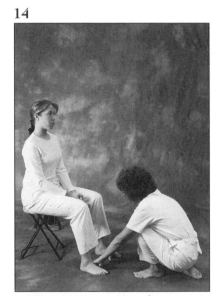

14: Practitioner opening the patient's feet and balancing the energy flow.

15

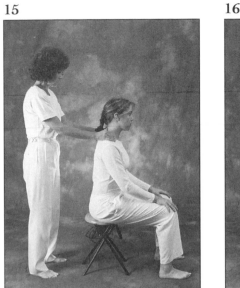

16

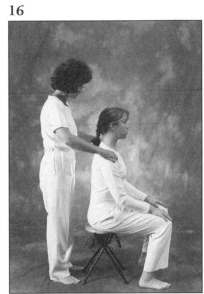

15-18: Practitioner opening the shoulders and directing energy flow down each arm (same procedure as opening the feet).

17

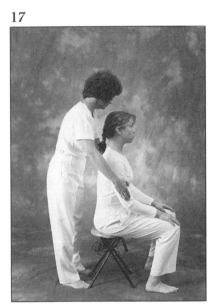

18

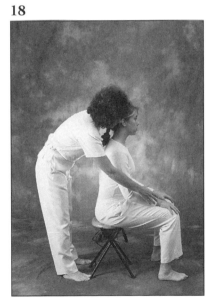

At this point in the treatment, the practitioner needs to perform another assessment, which can be done by repeating steps 7-11, and any appropriate intervention as described in chapter 7. The practitioner should also periodically check the patient's feet (step 14) to make sure they are open.

19

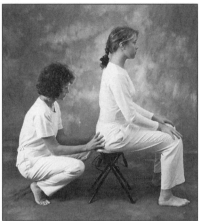

20

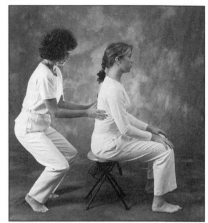

19: Practitioner gently moving down the patient's spine.

20: Practitioner building the energy ball to raise the life force, or Qi.

21

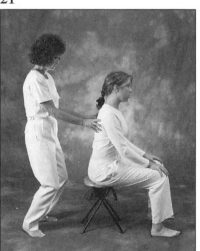

22

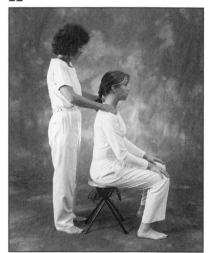

21-22: Practitioner slowly moving up the patient's spine while visualizing the energy ball, clearing the central tube, and raising the patient's energy.

23

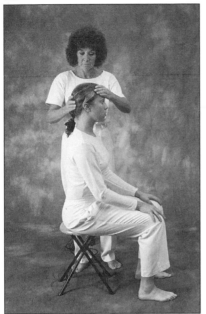

24

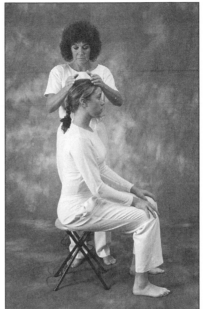

23-26: Practitioner releasing energy.

25

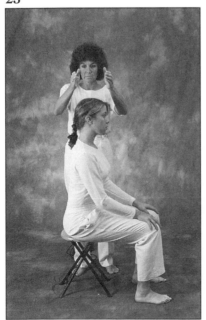

26

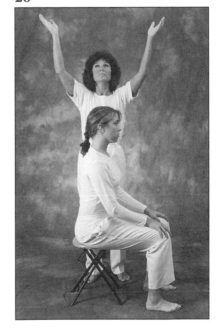

27

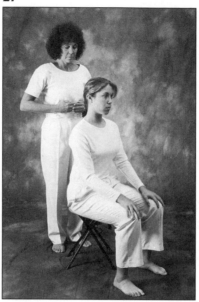

27: Practitioner returning light and
love to the patient's vibral core.

28

29

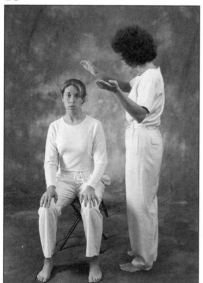
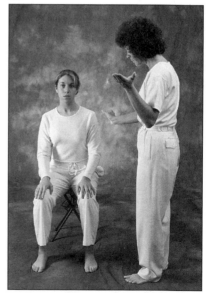

28-32: Practitioner grooming the field in a clockwise direction at the patient's
left side.

30

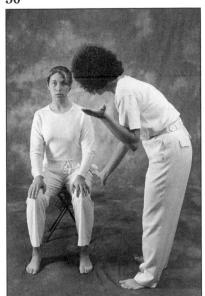

31

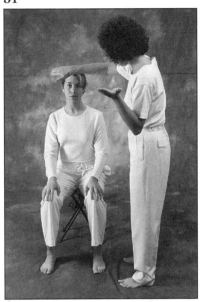

32

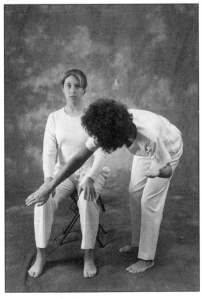

Balancing the Chakras with the Patient in a Supine or Lying-Down Position.

Complete treatment may also be given this way.

1

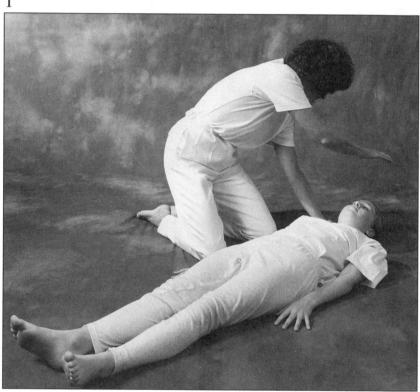

1-3: Initial assessment with the practitioner's left hand supporting the patient at the back of the neck.

2

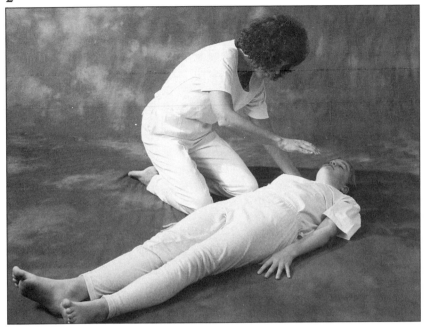

3

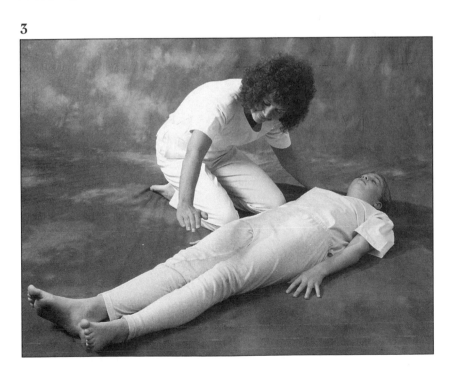

4

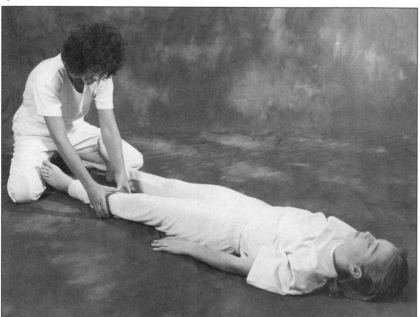

4-6: Practitioner pulling energy down both legs.

5

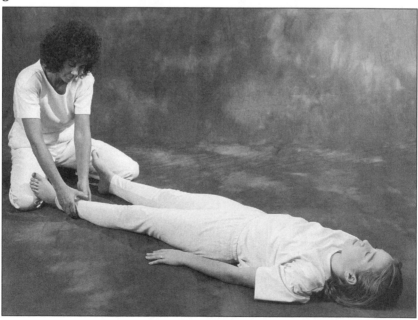

6

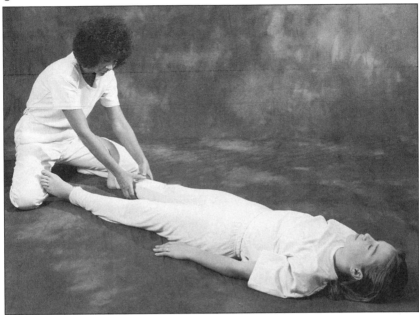

7

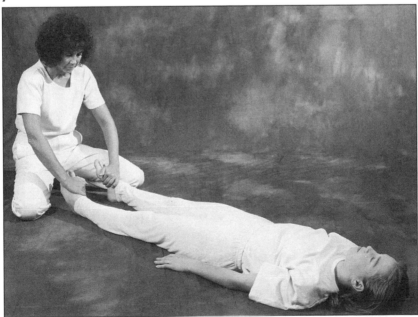

7: Practitioner opening the feet.

8

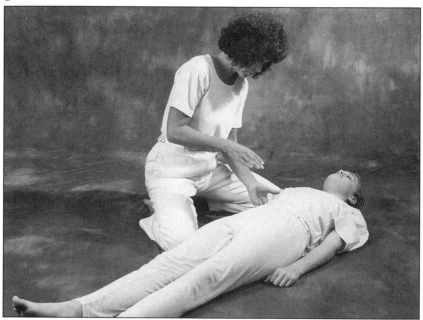

8-9: Practitioner placing hands around the patient's solar plexus.

9

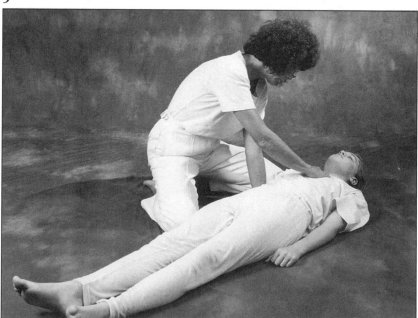

10

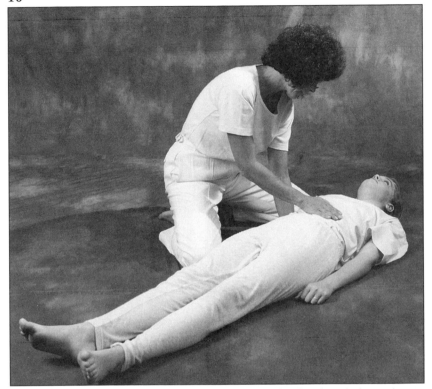

10: Practitioner visualizing the energy ball between her hands to balance the Chakra.

NOTE: The pictures depict only the solar plexus, but steps 8-10 may be done for any of the Chakras.

References

Berger, Ruth. *The Secret Is in the Rainbow*. York Beach, Maine: Samuel Weiser, Inc., 1979.

Berkow, Robert, M.D., ed. *Merck Manual of Diagnosis and Therapy*. 14th ed. Rahway, N.J.: Merck, Sharp, and Dohme Research Labs, 1982.

Besant, Annie, and Leadbeater, C. W. *Human Thought Forms*. Wheaton, Ill.: Theosophical Publishing House, 1969.

Boyde, William. *Textbook of Pathology*. 8th ed. Philadelphia: Lea and Febejer, 1970.

Brennan, Barbara A. *Hands of Light: A Healing Guide Through the Human Energy Field*. New York: Bantam Books, 1988.

Caine, Randy, and Bufalino, Patricia, eds. *Nursing Care Planning Guides for Adults*. Baltimore: Williams and Wilkins, 1987.

Chia, Mantah. *Awaken Healing Energy Through the Tao*. Santa Fe, N.M.: Aurora Press, 1983.

Chopra, Deepak, M.D. *Quantum Healing: Exploring the Frontiers of Mind/Body Medicine*. New York: Bantam Books, 1989.

Clark, P. E., and Clark, M. J. "Therapeutic Touch: Is There a Scientific Basis for the Practice?" *Nursing Research* 33(1) (1984):37–41.

Cooke, Ivan. *Healing by the Spirit*. Oxford, England: University Printing House, 1988.

Dolan, Marion. *Community & Home Health Care Plans*. Pa.: Springhouse Corporation, 1990.

Earl, Jonathan. "Cerebral Laterality and Meditation: A Review of the Literature." *Journal of Transpersonal Psychology* 13 (1981):155–73.

Fanslow, Cathleen A., R.N., M.A. "Therapeutic Touch: A Healing Modality Throughout Life." *Topics in Clinical Nursing* 5(2) (1983):72–79.

Fastwolf, Oh Shinnah. Various lectures on healing with crystals.

Gerber, Richard, M.D. *Vibrational Medicine.* Santa Fe, N.M.: Bear and Company, 1988.

Grad, Bernard. "The Influence of an Unorthodox Method of Wound Healing in Mice." *International Journal of Parapsychology,* Spring 1961, pp. 5–24.

———. "Some Biological Effects of 'Laying On of Hands': A Review of Experiments with Animals and Plants." *Journal of the American Society for Psychical Research* 59(2) (1965):95–127.

Heidt, Patricia, Ph.D., R.N. "Effect of Therapeutic Touch on Anxiety Level of Hospitalized Patients." *Nursing Research* 30(1) (1981):32–37.

Johari, Harish. *Chakras.* Rochester, Vt.: Destiny Books, 1987.

Judith, Anodea. *Wheels of Life.* St. Paul, Minn.: Llewellyn Publications, 1990.

Kaptchuk, Ted J. *The Web That Has No Weaver.* New York: Congdon and Weed, 1983.

Karagulla, Shafica, M.D., and van Gelder Kunz, Dora. *The Chakras.* Wheaton, Ill.: Theosophical Publishing House, 1989.

Kilner, Walter J. *The Human Aura.* Secaucus, N.J.: Citadel Press, 1965.

Krieger, Dolores, Ph.D., R.N. *Living the Therapeutic Touch: Healing as a Lifestyle.* New York: Dodd, Mead and Company, 1987.

———. *The Therapeutic Touch: How to Use Your Hands to Help and to Heal.* Englewood Cliffs, N.J.: Prentice-Hall, 1979.

———. "Therapeutic Touch: The Imprimatur of Nursing." *American Journal of Nursing* 5 (1975):784–87.

Krieger, Dolores, Ph.D., R.N., et. al. "Therapeutic Touch: Searching for Evidence of Physiological Change." *American Journal of Nursing,* April 1979, pp. 660–62.

Kunz, Dora, comp. *Spiritual Aspects of the Healing Arts.* Wheaton, Ill.: Theosophical Publishing House, 1985.

Landsdowne, Zachary, Ph.D. *The Chakras and Esoteric Healing.* York Beach, Maine: Samuel Weiser, Inc., 1986.

Laurie, Sanders G., and Tucker, Melvin J. *Centering: A Guide to Inner Growth.* Rochester, Vt.: Destiny Books, 1983.

Leadbetter, C. W. *The Chakras.* Wheaton, Ill.: Theosophical Publishing House, 1987.

Macrae, Janet. *Therapeutic Touch: A Practical Guide.* New York: Alfred A. Knopf, 1988.

———. "Therapeutic Touch in Practice." *American Journal of Nursing,* April 1979, pp. 664–65.

Miller, Lynn A. "An Explanation of Therapeutic Touch: Using the Science of Unitary Man." *Nursing Forum* 18(3) (1979):278–87.

Mitchell, Edgar D. *Psychic Exploration: A Challenge for Science.* New York: G. P. Putnam and Sons, 1974.

Nitsch, Twylah. Various lectures on healing.

O'Connor, John, and Bensky, Dan, trans. and eds. *Acupuncture: A Comprehensive Text.* Chicago: Eastland Press, 1981.

Pellitier, K. R. *Mind as Healer, Mind as Slayer.* New York: Dell Publishing, 1977.

Quinn, Janet, Ph.D., R.N. "One Nurse's Evolution as a Healer." *American Journal of Nursing,* April 1979, pp. 662–64.

Randolph, Gretchen L., Ph.D., R.N. "Therapeutic and Physical Touch: Physiological Response to Stressful Stimuli." *Nursing Research* 33(1) (1984):33–36.

Rea, John D. *Patterns of the Whole.* Vol. 1. Healing and Quartz Crystals. Boulder, Colo.: Two Trees Publishing, 1986.

Schwarz, Jack. *Human Energy Systems.* New York: E. P. Dutton, 1980.

———. *Voluntary Controls.* New York: E. P. Dutton, 1978.

Stein, Diane. *All Women Are Healers.* Calif.: Crossing Press, 1990.

———. *The Woman's Book of Healing.* St. Paul, Minn.: Llewellyn Publications, 1987.

Taber, Clarence Wilbur. *Taber's Cyclopedic Medical Dictionary.* 11th ed. Philadelphia: F. A. Davis Company, 1969.

Williams III, Gurney. "The Lowest-Tech Medicine Ever." *Longev-
    ity,* January 1992, pp. 60–69.
Wilson, Jean D., M.D., et al., eds. *Harrison's Principles of Internal
    Medicine.* 12th ed. New York: McGraw-Hill, Inc., 1991.

Resources Note

There is no national source list, as yet, for energy workers or Therapeutic Touch therapists. However, most cities have many people that are currently practicing. Places such as Interface in Cambridge, Massachusetts, or the Mind-Science Foundation in San Antonio, Texas, offer information and seminars about alternative healing practices. Some cities have a Holistic Healers Association, and usually local health food stores have an advertisement board where people who practice alternative healing will post their business cards.

Most major hospitals have nurses who practice energy work and Therapeutic Touch. The nursing department should have a list of those individual nurses.

There is also an organization called the American Holistic Nurses Association. Within this organization there is a group of people who teach classes on healing touch all over the country. The association is also an excellent source for individual practitioners. This information can be obtained by calling or writing to:

> Janet L. Mentgen, BSN, RN
> 198 Union Blvd.
> Suite 210
> Lakewood, CO 80725
> 303-989-0581

As time goes on and Therapeutic Touch becomes a more accepted adjunct to general medical practices, these listings will probably show up in the local yellow pages. Until then, however, you will have to do your own research to find them.

DEBY COWENS

Index

About the Author

Deborah Cowens is a nurse practitioner in women's health and a clinical specialist in psychiatry. For the past sixteen years she has had her own private practice, providing clients with physical exams, blood chemistry readings, nutritional supplement recommendations with dietary consultations, therapeutic touch, and guided imagery. She also worked with a gynecologist in Brookline, Massachusetts, doing annual exams, menopausal counseling, and colposcopic exams.

Cowens was also on the faculty at Regis College in Weston, Massachusetts, for six years. She has taught seminars at Interface, a holistic teaching center in Cambridge, Massachusetts, and has spoken before numerous organizations on topics ranging from nutrition to stress management. She also conducts a self-designed, ten-week course to teach nurses and other health care workers how to use therapeutic touch and energy work.

She currently resides in San Antonio, Texas, with her husband and two daughters.